MD/MBA: Physicians on the New Frontier of Medical Management

Edited by Arthur Lazarus, MD, MBA

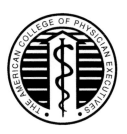

An ACPE Publication

ISBN: 0-924674-61-X
Library of Congress Card Number: 97-78156

Printed in the United States of America by Hillsborough Printing.

Contributors

Spencer Borden, IV, MD, MBA
Principal, Integrity Consulting, Inc., Concord, Massachusetts

David J. Brailer, MD, PhD
Chief Executive Officer, Care Management Science Corporation, The Wharton School, University of Pennsylvania, Philadelphia, Pennsylvania; Clinical Associate Professor of Medicine, University of Pennsylvania School of Medicine, Philadelphia, Pennsylvania

Wesley Curry
Managing Editor, Book Publishing, American College of Physician Executives, Tampa, Florida

Adele C. Foley, MA, MBA
Associate Dean and Director of MBA Programs, Graduate Business Office, St. Joseph's University, Philadelphia, Pennsylvania

Jennifer R. Grebenschikoff
Vice President, Physician Executive Management Center, Tampa, Florida

Howard J. Horwitz
Director of Professional Development, American College of Physician Executives, Tampa, Florida

Arthur Lazarus, MD, MBA
Medical Director, Behavorial Health Medicine, Prudential Healthcare, Horsham, Pennsylvania; Professor of Psychiatry, MCP/Hahnemann School of Medicine, Allegheny University of the Health Sciences, Philadelphia, Pennsylvania

John S. Lloyd, MBA, MPH
Vice Chairman, Witt/Kieffer, Ford, Hadelman, and Lloyd, Oak Brook, Illinois

Mary Frances Lyons, MD
Senior Consultant, Witt/Kieffer, Ford, Hadelman, and Lloyd, St. Louis, Missouri

David B. Nash, MD, MBA, FACPE
Associate Dean of Health Policy and Director, Office of Health Policy and Clinical Outcomes, Thomas Jefferson University Hospital, Philadelphia, Pennsylvania; Associate Professor of Medicine, Jefferson Medical College, Philadelphia, Pennsylvania

Ruth Pagano, MD, MBA, FACPE
Senior Medical Director, Anthem Blue Cross Blue Shield of Connecticut, North Haven, Connecticut

Geoffrey C. Porges, MBBS, MBA
Vice President, Worldwide Marketing Planning, Merck Vaccine Division, Merck & Company, West Point, Pennsylvania

Marshall de Graffenried Ruffin Jr., MD, MPH, MBA, FACPE
President, The Informatics Institute, Bethesda, Maryland

Joel I. Shalowitz, MD, MM
Professor and Program Director, Health Services Management Program, J.L. Kellogg Graduate School of Management, Northwestern University, Evanston, Illinois

Deborah M. Shlian, MD, MBA
Chief Executive Officer, Shlian and Associates, Inc., Boca Raton, Florida

Peter L. Slavin, MD, MBA
President, Barnes-Jewish Hospital, and Senior Executive Officer, Central Region, BJC Health System, St. Louis, Missouri.

James J. Unland, MBA
President, The Health Capital Group, Chicago, Illinois

David Whitehouse, MD, MBA, ThD
Senior Vice President and Corporate Medical Director, MCC Behavioral Care, Eden Prairie, Minnesota

George W. Winter, MA
Program Associate, MBA Managerial Communication Program, Curtis L. Carlson School of Management, University of Minnesota-Twin Cities, Minneapolis, Minnesota; Principal, Winter Communication, Saint Paul, Minnesota

Ronald N. Yeaple, PhD
Executive Professor of Business Administration, William E. Simon Graduate School of Business Administration, University of Rochester, Rochester, New York

Preface

As for-profit health care pushes physicians into the unfamiliar terrain of business and the reality of limited resources affects clinical practice, many physicians have begun to reevaluate their professional standing and career decisions. The ingredients required for success in business and in medicine have been changing over the past two decades in very important ways. Career paths and approaches to work that were previously effective are no longer paying dividends. Perhaps this is because careers today are less linear, more dynamic, and more unpredictable than mid-20th Century norms. Nevertheless, significant numbers of physicians are still trying to use old strategies to resolve contemporary problems wrought by the "crisis" in health care.

Career pathways in medicine—and in medical management in particular—have rarely been discussed openly. Yet this career path is gaining ground. In a survey conducted in 1994, nearly 10 percent of physicians in management jobs had MBAs, up from 6 percent in 1990 and virtually none in 1979. Another 38 percent of physicians said they were working on an MBA or intend to pursue one. It is a sign of the times that today's prestigious dual degree is the MD, MBA, not the esteemed MD, PhD, of yesteryear.

Physicians in the process of choosing medical management as a specialty need information about themselves and their options in order to make informed decisions. *MD/MBA: Physicians on the New Frontier of Medical Management* offers physicians guidance in assessing professional and personal strengths, developing self-marketing strategies, identifying and evaluating alternatives to conventional practice, and approaching career transitions in an organized way. In seeking such advice myself, I realized how little information existed and how useful a book like this could be for medical students, residents, and physicians at any stage in their careers.

The introductory chapter provides an overview of the medical management field and addresses such important questions as: What accounts for the recent influx of physicians into management? What types of management positions are within reach? When is the best time to obtain a graduate business degree? Which skills are necessary to navigate in the management arena? What barriers prevent physicians from achieving managerial effectiveness? The premise is that physician leaders who are fluent in both the business and the clinical aspects of health care will drive the reengineering process to reduce costs and improve outcomes.

The next several chapters deal specifically with the expectations of physicians in business school. Does it pay to get an MBA degree? What types of MBA programs can physicians choose from and what are the advantages and disadvantages of each? Do physicians with MBA degrees value them and recommend them to others? In Chapter 4, I have recounted my own experience in business school for those considering taking the plunge.

Business cynicism abounds despite a renaissance in MBA hiring throughout the country. Physicians duty-bound to the calling of management will be questioned by physicians and nonphysicians alike. Clearly, administration is not the panacea for unhappy or threatened clinicians. It is, however, a logical choice for physicians who want to influence the way health care is delivered by bringing a medical perspective to the business side of the industry.

Nowhere is this more evident than in the reflections of nine well-known physicians with MBA degrees whose careers are described in detail in Section 2. Autobiographical accounts of these physicians describe opportunities, challenges, and surprises as they progressed through the management ranks. Modern options in medical management are explored in light of health care reform and other forces affecting the practice of medicine. In this section we hear from a medical school dean, a health care consultant, a pharmaceutical company marketing executive, a health policy and clinical outcomes researcher, a managed behavioral healthcare executive, an information systems specialist, an insurance company medical director, a management search firm CEO, and a hospital senior vice president and chief medical officer. A wide range of career pathways in medical management awaits physicians who have the proper talent and credentials.

The last section of the book focuses on the physician as chief executive officer. The term "physician executive" is no longer an oxymoron. Many different types of health care organizations are benefiting from this new cadre of physicians who are more willing and able to join the ranks of senior management: hospitals and health networks, academic medical centers, and private industry, to name a few. A chapter on the career marketplace for physician executives is followed by one that depicts the road to the top as seen through the eyes of six physician CEOs. Chapters in this section also contain practical information for aspiring physician executives—for example, resources available thorough the American College of Physician Executives and a brief annotated reading list in medical management. The evolution of provider networks across the continuum of risk and the emergence of providers as insurers in their own right is discussed at length. Physicians empowered as chief executives are regaining control of health care for themselves, their colleagues, and the communities they serve.

Arthur Lazarus, MD, MBA
April 1998

Table of Contents

Section 3 143
The Physician Executive: Regaining Control of Health Care

Introduction ▬▬▬▬▬▬▬▬▬▬▬▬▬

The Management Challenge

by Joel I. Shalowitz, MD, MM

Over the past 10 to 15 years, challenges to physicians' professional and economic autonomy have multiplied and are occurring at an accelerated pace. While the apparent current culprit is managed care, in all its actual and imaginary forms, one can find the origins for these challenges in the recent and remote past. Rather than looking for excuses and scapegoats for the problems of our profession, many physicians are trying to regain some control by assuming managerial roles in an ever-increasing variety of health care-related organizations. While it is commonplace for physicians to be presidents of medical groups or department chairs in academic settings, it was not as common until recently for physicians to become health system CEOs or pharmaceutical company executives. Furthermore, few clinicians found their way to the top ranks of management consulting, and any representation in venture capital realms was rare. Frequently, physicians have replaced nonphysicians in these management roles. In entering these positions, physicians need to extend their skills to such areas as marketing, strategic positioning, information systems design, and mergers and acquisitions. Even in their traditional roles, physicians' responsibilities are becoming less clinical and more managerial. Without further training, however, we can never achieve professional parity with those whose jobs have historically been in health care management.

Given the current status of the profession, the questions that naturally arise are: How did we get here? Why are physicians entering management careers in unprecedented numbers? What career paths can we expect to follow? How can we best prepare ourselves to meet the challenges of these roles? What are some of the obstacles we face? What does the future hold? I shall attempt to answer these questions below.

How Did We Get Here?

The current growing scrutiny of the medical profession is not a recent phenomenon. In fact, it is not entirely due to managed care. Its origins are ancient and derive from patients' expectations of our capabilities, many of which we created. In ancient cultures, we were religious and/or secular leaders. We were called Imhotep, Aesclepius, shaman, and king. At the very time when we could do the least, we were held in the highest regard by our patients. If they did not recover, it was the will of the gods, not the fault of physicians. While the Renaissance brought a greater knowledge of medicine, particularly anatomy and physiology, our capabilities to treat illness did not keep pace. We pretended, however, that it did. The public became aware of the fallibility of the profession, and parodies such as those of Molière clearly and bluntly reflected those views. By the middle to late 19th Century, we knew more about the epidemiology of some diseases and, in some cases, even its prevention. Treatments, however, still remained relatively primitive. Further, hospitals continued to be places where the dying went as a refuge of last resort, not a place of salvation from a variety of afflictions. It is important to note that many hospitals were still run by religious orders, continuing the ancient tradition linking medicine and religion.

The first modern watershed for the profession occurred at the beginning of the 20th Century, particularly with capabilities in surgery. We were able to safely anesthetize a patient, perform surgery with relatively low rates of infection, and transfuse blood, if needed. Testing also became more sophisticated, particularly serology and radiology. The natural place for these sophisticated services was the hospital, and its natural leader was often a physician In fact, in many countries today, e.g., Japan, physicians are the only professionals allowed to run hospitals. Reimbursement was simple then. If one could afford to pay for treatment, the payment was in cash. If such payment was not forthcoming, many institutions delivered care as part of their mission of community service. Hospital trustees were financial benefactors of the institution who also determined who was admitted and treated.

The second watershed dates from the proliferation of commercial health insurance, particularly after World War II. This major change in reimbursement was accompanied by an acceleration in the development and implementation of technology. Along with these two significant transforming events came the origins of our current problems: unrestrained growth in technology and the unconditional promise to pay for it. These two issues have continued to feed on one another to the present: the more medicine can do, the more the public expects and the more it wants covered by health policies. (Witness, for example, such state mandates for health insurance as *in vitro* fertilization.) Further, evaluation of the efficacy of much of this technology awaited the growth of managed care plans. While physicians would not knowingly harm a patient by doing more tests, performing more surgery, or prescribing medication, practice patterns were often dictated by what seemed logical rather than what was known from controlled studies. Management of institutions with more complex reimbursement and technology required professionals formally trained in the business aspects of health care. It is no coincidence that the first graduate programs in this discipline were founded during this period. (The two oldest programs in health care management are at the University of Chicago and at Northwestern University, which were started in 1939 and 1943, respectively.) While many of these programs were started by, or with aid from, physicians, most of the graduates did not have medical training. Hospital management, therefore, rapidly became the province of nonclinicians. Likewise, while some pharmaceutical companies (e.g., Abbott) were started by physicians, control was shortly turned over to professionally trained managers.

The third watershed occurred in 1966, with implementation of Medicare and Medicaid. That event marked the entry of government, particularly the federal government, into significant involvement in the health insurance business. In order to curb rapidly rising hospital expenses, Medicare shifted from a cost-plus basis, to a cost-basis, to a diagnosis-related group method of payment. Likewise, it changed payment for physician services from a customary, prevailing, and reasonable schedule (with all the problems of the private sector's usual, customary, and reasonable method of payment) to a geography-based fee schedule that it claimed was resource-based (the resource-based relative value scale, or RBRVS). While some look to government programs as relief from managed care inroads, these payment changes have, in fact, fueled the growth of managed care plans. With the advent of DRGs, hospitals accelerated their search for ways to make up lost income— euphemistically called "cost shifting." The obvious source was raising the rates paid by commercial insurers, many of whom were still paying full charges. In order to cover these rapidly rising costs, insurers passed along the expense in the form of higher premiums to their customers. After years of double-digit rises in these premiums (the cost of which sometimes equaled companies' net profits), corporate America demanded more cost-accountability in the insurance products it purchased. By 1992, the majority of health insurance plans purchased by corporations were health maintenance organization (HMO), preferred provider organization (PPO), or point of service (POS) products. Per diem charges are now the predominant way these plans pay for hospital care. When not employing capitation, many private plans have followed the federal cost-containment lead in paying physicians using fee schedules based on RBRVS.

A fourth watershed emerged from the consumer and individual rights movements, which started to flourish in the 1960s. Individuals began to ask more questions about the products and services they purchased or used and demanded data for comparison shopping. Health care was no exception. Women, in particular, were learning to challenge the paternalistic nature of medicine. They started to ask questions about such procedures as hysterectomies, as well as about alternatives to radical mastectomies for breast cancer. Consumer activists challenged a system in which the more that was done, the more someone else paid. These same consumers, and their larger group of disciples, are also concerned about capitated systems where, apparently, the less one does the more one gets paid.

Why Physicians Are Interested in Management

Physicians who are interested in management have stepped into this environment in increasing numbers over the past decade. From numerous interviews conducted during that time, I have found that they have several reasons for wanting to obtain formal management training. First, many want to "retool" for another career in health care. Often, these positions are removed from direct patient care—e.g., medical director of a managed care plan. Occasionally, the jobs combine clinical responsibilities with management duties—e.g., section chief or department chair in an academic setting. Second, some physicians wish to advance in their current career pathway but are unable to do so without formal management training. Again, academic positions are starting to fall into this category. Third, some are finding that their current jobs require additional skills for which they were not formally trained. In addition to the positions mentioned above, one could add Vice President of Medical Affairs (or a similar title) for a hospital or organized delivery system.

Fourth, a small, but growing number of physicians are either tired of patient care or never had any intention of making that aspect of the profession their lives' work. These physicians enter management school with the aim of obtaining the same credentials as their "MBA colleagues" and of competing with them for the same jobs. These jobs may or may not have anything to do with the direct provision of health care. An example of such a field, which is growing in popularity, is venture capital. Physicians who enter these careers are different from the others mentioned above, because they are really "MBAs with MDs" rather than "MDs with MBAs." The final major reason given by applicants to management school is one of default. They are tired of their current careers, or the path medical practice has taken, and look to management as an easy alternative. Their time would be better spent with a career counselor than an admissions officer. Their lack of purpose will be detected by any top school and their likelihood of admission is slim.

Typical Career Paths

Given these reasons for seeking management training, the skills one needs to acquire will vary, depending on a number of factors: into which of the above five categories the physician falls, the desired type of organization for whom he or she will work, personal interest and ability, and job entry level. While it is beyond the scope of this introduction to list all the combinations of job types, firms, and personal interests, a general overview of skills needed at each career stage will be presented. Although these stages can often seamlessly flow into one another, for discussion purposes it is useful to separate them into three levels.

The first stage is an entry-level position. While the descriptions and titles of these jobs will vary by type of organization, what they all share is the requirement that *you* do the work. Examples range from budget preparation to marketing surveys to research reports in specific functional areas. The required skills are therefore task-oriented. Knowledge of accounting and financial reporting, marketing, and statistical methods are only some of the types of proficiencies that one must bring to an entry-level position.

In the second stage, one starts to become a true manager. The feature distinguishing this stage from the previous one is budgetary authority and the ability to hire and fire personnel. (These are the same distinctions that differentiate line from staff positions in organizations.) Knowledge about the output of entry-level personnel, while necessary, is not sufficient. Managers must also be adept at integrating multiple sources of information, perceiving trends, and making appropriate resource allocations. Further skills one must have are the ability to foster team building and to develop a highly functioning organizational culture. I believe that these latter skills, if successfully applied, will give any organization a sustainable competitive advantage.

The final stage is "top management," where one has responsibility for a substantial portion, if not all, of the enterprise. Building on the previous skill set, one needs to enhance negotiation skills, for use both inside and outside the organization; foster system thinking throughout the firm; and develop what has become known as a "learning organization," i.e., help the enterprise continuously learn from its successes and mistakes and improve on the basis of those experiences. At the highest levels of this stage are those who are in positions to shape public policy through their knowledge and/or political contacts. In these cases, experience with government politics, coalition building, and business ethics are called into play and are rigorously tested.

It should be noted that one cannot learn or master all these skills even in a master's degree curriculum. There is not enough time and the tasks one is expected to perform on graduation usually do not require proficiency in all areas. What this statement implies is that, like medicine, management education is a lifelong learning process. Not only do theories and tools change, but also the appropriate ones for different career stages evolve. One must, therefore, continue to read and attend courses to acquire new skills and hone existing ones.

Suggested Educational Pathways

The question that logically follows is: What is the best venue for acquiring these skills? In answering this question, one can first divide curricula between short course programs and formal degree training. The former can range from single topics (such as "Finance for Nonfinancial Managers") lasting days to a series of topics (such as those offered by the American College of Physician Executives) that can take many weeks to complete. The advantages of such courses are that they are short, easy to schedule, cost relatively little, and give a desired sampling of management topics. The disadvantage is that they do not provide the depth and scope of a full degree curriculum. They also often focus only on health care issues, missing the richness of examples and best practices offered by other industries.

Formal degree training can be categorized by the types of degrees offered. Before the past decade, a common additional graduate degree for physicians was the master of public health (MPH). Although this degree continues to be appropriate for those who wish to pursue careers in such disciplines as epidemiology, the skills taught in such programs are often not applicable to a wide variety of management positions. For example, it is unlikely that an investment banking firm seeking a financial analyst or a medical product firm looking for a brand manager would initially consider a candidate with a public health degree.

A more management-related degree is the master in health care administration (MHA). This degree was the traditional one for hospital administrators for many years. Because many physicians view this degree as a natural extension of medicine into business, it has become a popular choice for graduate study. Many of these programs, however, have been undergoing a philosophic change in the past five years. Their educational orientation was to teach health care primarily and bring business concepts into the curriculum as needed. As a result of a desire to have a more business focus, a number of MHA programs have either moved into their universities' business schools, e.g., Duke, or established joint degree programs with those schools, e.g., University of Michigan. By contrast, the model at Northwestern University has been full integration into the school of management for more than 20 years. MHA degrees are still appropriate choices for many physicians seeking opportunities in traditional health care careers.

Physicians' choice of a business school curriculum has become increasingly popular over the past 10 years and is the thrust of this book. The primary reasons for the choice are the diversity of career options that have become available and the more numerous and varied skills required to manage increasingly complex health care organizations. Some of these positions, such as management consulting and pharmaceutical company management, have been recently occupied by nonphysicians. A growing number of careers are becoming available for former clinicians in fields not usually associated with health care, e.g., venture capital and investment banking, as mentioned above. Physicians who want to expand their possibilities for employment and who see "MBAs" as their competitors for these jobs will opt for the management degree over an MHA or MPH.

The advantages of degree programs over short courses are the extent of training and the credibility they bring to the job market. The disadvantages are the time it takes to complete the curriculum and the associated nominal and opportunity costs. The overall trend, however, is for physicians to obtain management degrees if they anticipate career changes into administration rather than a modification of their current positions. It is also important to note that while, in the short run, certification in medical management serves a useful function in helping the marketplace sort out the various credentials of clinicians-turned-managers, as more physicians earn degrees from leading graduate schools, such certification may become moot. I have never heard of any firm asking graduates of top management schools whether or not they were certified in medical management or intended to become certified.

Timing of Graduate Education

In light of these training options, when is the best time to obtain a graduate degree? Seven career stages can be identified at which physicians may seek this option. The advantages and disadvantages of graduate studies at each stage will be briefly discussed below.

The first stage is during medical school. In a growing number of formal joint MD/MBA programs, students can complete both curricula in five years instead of the traditional six. The advantage at this stage is that the additional education is part of continuous schooling and students are still used to heavy academic workloads. The disadvantages are assumption of additional debt (when the burden may already be substantial) and the fact that the management skills that they learn will not be used until several years after graduation. As is the case with medical learning, one must use management knowledge to remain proficient. Since the establishment of the MD/MM program at Northwestern more than 10 years ago, however, I have not observed graduates having any of these difficulties.

The second stage occurs immediately after medical school. At this point, it is common to find physicians from foreign countries, where residencies are not necessarily routine. Because of the lack of uniformity in postgraduate training abroad, international medical graduates who only complete medical school are often perceived as peers by their fellow physicians in their countries. Furthermore, because physicians who obtain formal management degrees abroad are rare, they are distinguished by the additional training. In this country, however, physicians are not credible with their colleagues unless they have comparable clinical credentials and, in many cases, continue to see patients. This credibility factor makes it critical for U.S. medical school graduates to complete residencies and achieve board certification, even if they have no intention of providing direct patient care. The one exception would be those planning careers in bench research.

The third stage is during residency. It is difficult to integrate this training with many residency programs, such as surgery, where the call is frequent and residents have significant ongoing patient care responsibilities. Some specialties, e.g., pathology, in which the hours are more predictable would lend themselves to pursuing a graduate management degree. Formal training programs in this stage are rare.

The fourth stage occurs immediately after residency. Family and professional commitments are relatively few, although loan payments from college and medical school often start to become due. The students I have seen at this stage, however, usually do not encounter academic or financial hardship. Clinical moonlighting jobs often help defray educational costs and living expenses, while keeping medical skills somewhat intact.

The fifth stage is early career, which I define as up to five years after residency. Time here is spent building a practice and demonstrating to peers one's profitability, productivity, and proficiency. If one is in a physician-owned practice, this time is important in demonstrating the potential for partnership. Add to these barriers the disadvantages of post-residency time mentioned above, and it is clear this is not the best time to pursue a graduate degree.

The sixth stage is mid-career, which I define as five to 20 years post-residency, or from one's mid- to late thirties to one's late forties or early fifties. Practice experience begins to peak sometime during this period, and career goals often become clearer. On the downside, family commitments and financial responsibilities are usually the greatest, making opportunity costs highest at this stage. In the previous stages, full-time graduate work is an attractive option. During this stage, part-time study or executive programs become more appropriate.

The final stage is late-career. Financial stability is usually greatest at this stage, but the "return" on graduate degree education must be individually assessed. At this time, shorter courses become more appropriate than full degrees in order to fill gaps in experience. I anticipate that, in the next 10 to 15 years, MD/MBAs with moderate to significant work experience will fill the majority of high-profile management positions occupied by physicians. Late career practitioners without graduate degrees and experience will, therefore, not be able to easily compete in that market. This situation will particularly apply to such positions as Vice President for Medical Affairs. Currently, this job is, in many cases, occupied by respected late-career practitioners who do not possess formal management training but who can build consensus because of the high regard they enjoy from their colleagues.

Career Progress and Skills

In addition to formal management training, career advancement requires broad and credible practice and management experience. I advise those who are undergraduates or in medical school, who anticipate a career in medical management, and who have no preconceived specialty preferences to choose internal medicine or family practice as their specialty. The reason for this recommendation is that these specialties interface with the broadest complement of other medical disciplines; these practitioners are, therefore, more likely to understand a patient's needs from a variety of perspectives than, say, a surgical specialist. Pediatrics is also a good choice, but for a different reason. Good pediatricians always need to deal with families in the care of their patients. My experience has been that this perspective gives them a systems approach to care that other physicians may not have. Of more than parenthetical interest, it is also easier for primary care physicians than it is for other specialists to make the transition from clinical practice to management in terms of income differentials.

From a career development standpoint, one must consider the particular sector one wishes to enter. That said, I believe the best general training is currently in medical group management.

Some of the skills one must have to be successful in this arena are:

- Knowing about multiple forms of reimbursement, particularly such features of managed care plans as the actuarial basis and operational features of full-risk capitation, contracting, claims adjudication, utilization review, credentialing, and case management.

- Understanding principles, implementation, and evaluation of clinical and management quality improvement. Risk management is also included in this category.

- Grasping financial principles, including understanding financial statements, budgeting, making capital investment decisions, and managing cash flow.

- Learning how to employ situation-specific leadership and team building skills and to manage other professionals.

- Understanding personnel issues, such as incentive and bonus systems and benefit design and management—e.g., health insurance and pension/profit sharing.

- Being able to clearly communicate to internal and external constituencies such messages as organizational vision, mission, and reasons for policies and procedures.

- Being able to negotiate effectively with internal and external constituencies and to effectively resolve disputes. This resolution does not always mean a "win-win" situation.

Obstacles to Managerial Effectiveness

Once a physician has identified the format, timing, and necessary skills for a management career, at least three obstacles remain. The first impediment is external. The traditional management world often cannot accept a physician in any roles other than those pertaining to clinical care. Part of the problem may be analogous to "type casting" of character actors. While those who hire physician managers may need expertise with clinical areas, they cannot understand that these physicians may bring more to the team than that relatively narrow focus. For example, many major corporations do not involve their medical directors in the selection or design of medical benefits. One also cannot overlook the potential for jealousy; if physician managers possess skills in general management as well as in clinical areas, customers for their services may value them more highly than those without a medical background. The only way to overcome this obstacle is for physicians to obtain the same training and credentials as their managerial colleagues and prove to them on the job that they add significant value with their broad set of skills. In time, the mutual trust that is built will benefit both parties.

The second obstacle physician managers may encounter is narrow training in and thinking about health care-specific topics. Many degree and nondegree management education programs are geared specifically to the field. Also, by design, program attendees are all from the health care field. While this specificity is appropriate in some cases—e.g., accounting for health care organizations—physicians often miss out on the richness of the lessons that can be learned from "best of class" companies in other industries. Two of many relevant examples from other businesses include customer service (reservations, customer greeting, and recovery from service errors) and information system design and point of service data processing. One way to overcome this obstacle is to obtain a management degree along with classmates who come from different fields. Taking courses outside of health care is also essential to obtain this "out of the box" view. For short courses, I recommend taking some offerings geared primarily to managers from other fields. Courses do not need to have the words "in health care" appended to their titles to be useful. Explore such topics as sales force management, negotiations, and service quality and marketing.

The third obstacle is the result of typical medical training. As physicians, we are taught to care for patients one at a time and to be patients' advocates. Managers, on the other hand, are trained to look at the entire organization and determine what course of action is appropriate for it. While both responsibilities can be proper and laudatory, one needs to strike a balance between them. Physicians need to adopt a systems approach when acting as managers, never losing sight, however, that advocating for an individual may be the correct course of action in certain circumstances.

What May the Future Hold?

The responsibilities of physician managers only begin with educational training and job performance. In order to fulfill our obligation to society and resume a leadership role in the health care field, our profession must:

- Lobby for rational technology assessment policies and help introduce drugs, devices, and procedures that have demonstrated value to those we serve.

- Determine the most cost-effective ways to implement care across a continuum of services.

- Create realistic expectations about the outcomes of care for those who use or pay for our services (our "customers").

- Help return health insurance to the purpose for which it was originally intended—to indemnify against catastrophic loss. From there we can build a system of universal protection, as opposed to piecemeal coverage of conditions advocated by special interests.

- Deliver value to our customers, which I define as the best quality one can give for a specified price, or, for a desired level of quality, provide value at the lowest possible price. Delivering that value will require us to be able to measure and demonstrate quality in terms that our customers can understand. We must also be able to assess total costs per-case, as opposed to assigning prices to individual components of care. All of these capabilities will compel us to manage actual or virtually integrated systems.

- Lobby lawmakers to pass rational safeguards for our patients, not piece-meal restrictions that will inhibit the clinical and managerial aspects of delivering high-quality, efficient care.

I believe that, if we can obtain the training to allow us to accomplish these goals and avoid distracting and divisive interspecialty conflicts, we can resume our leadership position in the health care field and reclaim some of the professional and economic autonomy that we have recently lost.

Section 1
Business School:
A Traveler's Advisory

Chapter 1

Why It Pays to Get an MBA

by Ronald N. Yeaple, PhD

The Management Challenge in Health Care

Medicine has become a business—a highly competitive business—and even the most prestigious medical facilities are not exempt. For example, the *Wall Street Journal* recently described how New York's Memorial Sloan-Kettering Cancer Center, a world-class cancer center with a $1.4 billion endowment, has become embroiled in the same kind of struggle that has confronted much of the rest of American industry—fierce price competition, layoffs, closing of facilities, and early retirement of senior executives:

"Memorial Sloan-Kettering Cancer Center, one of the world's most prominent cancer facilities, finally yielded to the pressures of managed care. After months of secret negotiations, the center last week quietly signed a sweeping new contract with Empire Blue Cross and Blue Shield, New York state's largest health insurer. Under the contract, the cancer center will gain a flow of new patients in exchange for cutting its rates as much as 30%.

"...While operating at a loss in recent years, [Sloan-Kettering] has been tapping into revenue from donations and other sources. It wasn't enough. In the past three years, Sloan-Kettering closed three patient floors totaling 148 beds, or nearly a fourth of its total bed capacity. It has also laid off nurses and other staff and paid $8 million in early-retirement packages to 164 employees, including doctors and executives.

"The center's occupancy rate has hovered around 60%, according to New York State Health Department records. While it continues to be rated as the top cancer center in the nation, Sloan-Kettering has had difficulty adapting to the new environment brought about by the rise of health maintenance organizations."[1]

The Need for Professional Management

As health care continues to evolve as a highly competitive business, it demands professionally trained managers and leaders. Management can no longer succeed in running a health care organization by winging it on the basis of intuition and experience. Hard work, intelligence, and commitment are not enough. Today it takes professional training in the field of management.

What do managers have to know to be personally and professionally successful? For many years, businesses operated on the apprentice system. Young men and women joined a firm and were taught what they needed to know by their supervisors, just as novice silversmiths were apprenticed to master craftsmen at the time of Paul Revere. Business was seen as a trade rather than as a science. There was no agreed-upon body of knowledge for the conduct of a business.

Nowhere was this more apparent than in the universities. In the 1960s and '70s, while university research was ascending in importance in the health and physical sciences, the business schools of the time were under attack for being dull and unscientific. Looked upon with disdain by the "real scientists" on campus, business schools were often regarded as little more than trade schools, teaching case histories based on one-of-a-kind "war stories" that were of questionable generalizability to other business situations. Business was a course of study for students who couldn't make it in engineering or premed.

During this period, a few business schools, such as Chicago, MIT, and the University of Rochester, took a hard look at what was being taught and came up with sweeping changes. Business school professors who had undergraduate degrees in engineering as well as PhDs in economics set standards for the same rigorous analysis demanded in the physical sciences. By testing their theories in real management situations, these business school professors learned which theories were most useful for solving problems that managers face in the running of a business. And from this real-world experience came a common body of knowledge in various fields, such as finance and marketing, that eventually found its way into textbooks and classrooms. The practice of management was on its way to becoming less of a trade and more of a science.[2]

What Skills Do You Need to Succeed as a Manager?

Let's assume that you are considering a career in health care management. What are the critical management skills that you would need to achieve personal and professional success?

In the spring and summer of 1995, I conducted two comprehensive mail surveys of alumni of the Simon Graduate School of Business Administration and of the Department of Electrical Engineering, both at the University of Rochester. The objective of the study was to find out what management skills have been most valuable in contributing to respondents' personal and professional success.

A total of 550 questionnaires were mailed out to a random sample of Simon School alumni, all of whom have MBA degrees, and 273 usable responses were returned, for a response rate of 50 percent. Similarly, from a random sample of 500 electrical engineering alumni, I received 208 usable responses, for a response rate of 42 percent.

The ages of the respondents ranged from 22 to 73. Salaries ranged from graduate students scraping by on $10,000 per year to investment bankers earning $1 million a year. It was clear that most of the respondents took the survey seriously. Many filled the margins of the questionnaire with extra comments, and a few enclosed thoughtful letters full of advice for aspiring managers.[3]

In summarizing the data from the nearly 500 survey respondents, I learned that there were 10 strategic skills that were important to their success.[4]

Strategic Skill #1: Taking Charge as CEO of Your "Company of One"

Many of our survey respondents reported that the first step in becoming a successful manager is learning to manage one's self. The essence of many of their responses was: "Manage your own career...no one else will." "Learn to think of yourself as the CEO of a 'company of one'—yourself."

These managers and professionals reported that, in today's turbulent environment, you can't expect your organization to take care of you, even if you do excellent work. Only 22 percent of our respondents—the majority of whom are very successful—agreed with the statement, "If you do excellent work, you can trust your company to promote you." You cannot rely on your employer to manage your career. To succeed, you must develop a long-range personal strategy for your 'company of one.'

Strategic Skill #2: Obtaining General Business Knowledge

To succeed in any business, including the business of health care, you must understand how businesses work. If you intend to win, you must understand the rules of the game. According to our survey respondents, there are six basic areas in which general business knowledge is essential in achieving personal and professional success:

- *Cost Accounting*—not the most exciting area of study for most of us, but it is the language of business, the means by which your success is measured—and a treacherous minefield for the uninformed manager. You need a working knowledge of such cost accounting concepts as fixed versus variable costs, transfer prices, profit centers, absorption cost systems, straight line depreciation, and activity-based costing.

- *Financial accounting*—the means by which organizations disclose their financial condition to banks and owners, through quarterly and annual reports.

- *Microeconomics*—the basic science of business. Economics is to business as physics is to engineering.

- *Finance*—the most popular area of concentration in business school. Finance provides methods for evaluating alternative investment decisions under conditions of uncertainty, whether that investment is a new MRI machine for the clinic or new patient billing software for the office.

- *Marketing*—the way organizations reach out and serve their customers, who ultimately decide whether that organization stays in business.

- *Operations management*—the process by which the organization produces and delivers its goods and services to its customers. The goal of operations management is to produce and deliver the highest quality products and services in the shortest time, and at the lowest cost—essential in today's competitive health care industry.

Strategic Skill #3: Acquiring Specific Industry Knowledge

Everyone says it is important to understand your customers, but today you need more that that. You need to understand how your organization competes in its industry. To make the best decisions, you and your professional colleagues must understand your organization's overall strategy. If, for example, your organization's strategy is to be the lowest-cost, no-frills producer among the competitors who make up its market, the designs of the individual product and service offerings must reflect this strategy.

Strategic Skill #4: Sharpening Your Analytical Abilities

Some people think that business decisions can be based solely on common sense, intuition, and experience, but this is no longer true. The highest paid 10 percent of our research survey respondents—all making $200,000 or more—ranked analytical problem-solving skill as the most valuable area of competence for professionals and managers, based on their own career success.

Analytical skills are vitally important because managers are regularly called upon to make decisions under conditions of uncertainty—forecasts of next year's sales, estimated profitability of a proposed new product, or future returns on investment opportunities in the securities markets. Business has become too complex for you to succeed by "winging it." If you are not proficient with these analytical techniques, you will be outgunned by those in the marketplace who are.

The best decision-makers combine analytical skill with intuition and experience. Intuition includes the ability to discern complex patterns—based on years of experience—that are too subtle for formal analysis.

Strategic Skill #5: Building Computer Competence

Computers favor the young. Because young managers have grown up with computers, computer proficiency offers youth a huge advantage in the competition for good jobs. A journalist sitting in at a management meeting at Microsoft Corporation observed: "The oldest person in the room was 30; the rest were in their early 20s." Fifty-year-old managers are losing out, less because of age than because of obsolescence. Those that consider touching a keyboard to be secretarial work are at most risk.

According to our research survey, 95 percent of all managers have a computer in their offices, and they are more than just fancy typewriters—88 percent reported using spreadsheet applications within the past month. Whatever else you do in developing your strategic skills, don't back away from computers. Remember, it is obsolete managers who get the pink slips in a corporate downsizing.

Strategic Skill #6: Learning to Manage Innovation

Innovation is the great driving engine of our economy. Huge personal fortunes have been built by innovators such as Microsoft founder Bill Gates. As our survey showed, 95 percent of managers have PCs in their offices, and yet the PC is little more than a decade-and-a-half old. Medicine is being revolutionized by innovations such as MRI machines and genetic engineering. Automobiles have been transformed by dozen of embedded microprocessors and telecommunications by cellular telephones and the Internet.

Not all business innovations are the result of breakthrough technologies. In retailing, Sam Walton created Wal-Mart, envisioning a new approach to distribution featuring high-quality merchandise, low prices, and friendly and knowledgeable personal service. Michael Dell saw the potential for mail-order distribution of personal computers that bypassed traditional PC dealers and built a multibillion dollar company. In the field of innovative services, Fred Smith conceived an overnight package delivery service that became FedEx.

If innovation is a good strategy for corporations, would it not also be a good strategy for your personal "company of one?" The answer is yes, but you must address the following issues first:

- How do you go about changing the dominant thinking in your organization—or can you? Remember that large organizations—and the individuals who run them—have a major stake in keeping things as they are.

- Innovation is risky. It is said that success has many fathers, but failure is an orphan. What steps can you take to protect yourself by reducing this risk?

- How do you get credit for your innovations?

Strategic Skill #7: Developing Skills for Working with People

People skills—the ability to get things done through other people—are what distinguish managers from individual contributors. People skills include leadership, teamwork, and the ability to persuade others through written and oral communications.

Learning to lead and to manage people are perhaps the most difficult of the strategic skills to acquire. In our survey of business school graduates, the respondents agreed that, while MBA programs do a great job of teaching analytical skills, they are weak in teaching people skills. As one plant engineer who graduated with an MBA in 1983 wrote on his survey: "Technical knowledge is good, but people and managerial skills make the executive."

With the decline of organizational hierarchy, interpersonal relationships are based less on authority of command and more on cooperative associations of peers—task forces, multidisciplinary new product development teams—that are much like strategic alliances between companies. In today's organizations, with the relaxing of formal organizational structures, people skills are more important for the success of your "company of one" than ever before. You must learn to persuade people to do things—not because you are the boss, but because your ideas make sense for the organization.

Strategic Skill #8: Polishing Your Personal Core Competencies

Core competencies are the cornerstone of your personal strategy. Personal core competencies are the things you do for your organization that clearly set you apart from others—skills that make you special and exceptionally valuable to your employer. An example of a corporate core competency is 3M's world-class technology to put coatings of different substances on various kinds of substrates—sandpaper, magnetic tape, Post-It Notes, Scotch tape, reflective highway signs, and computer diskettes.

Examples of personal core competencies might include your knowledge of how to design new medical instruments, your special language skills that make you valuable in treating patients from foreign countries, or your in-depth knowledge of certain parts of the tax code to save your organization thousands of dollars every year.

But before you invest time developing your own personal core competencies, there are some important questions you need to consider. For example, what steps can you take to ensure that your core competencies will add real value to your organization? How will you participate in the rewards from mastering these core competencies? And how do you avoid their becoming obsolete?

Strategic Skill #9: Learning to Market Yourself

To get the highest return from your investment in your strategic skills, people who would value these skills have to be made aware of them. As our research survey respondents made emphatically clear, the premise that you will get promoted if you just do a good job is, unfortunately, naïve. As CEO of your "company of one," you must learn to market your strategic skills within your organization and on the outside, among those in your professional field.

Marketing your "company of one" is more than just selling yourself. You need a marketing plan. You must decide what the goal of your marketing effort is. You need to decide who your target audience is and what message you want to deliver. And you need to determine the best media for delivering that message and the optimal timing of the message.

Strategic Skill #10: Selecting and Cultivating a Board of Mentors

Mentors are a board of directors for your "company of one." In our research study, respondents reported that help and advice from senior managers who served as mentors was as valuable to their professional success as the content of the MBA courses they took.

Successful mentoring relationships don't just happen—they have to be developed and managed. Moreover, in today's complex organizations, you need more that just one mentor. You should aim to have a group of mentors with differing skills and positions both inside and outside the firm to serve as a board of directors for your "company of one."

In selecting your board of mentors, consider the following candidates:

- *Your boss* (ex officio). Like it or not, your boss is a member of your board of mentors by virtue of his or her power over your future.

- *Another senior manager* (but not your boss's boss or one of your boss's enemies). This mentor can give you a wider picture of what is happening in the organization, and he or she may be able to tip you off about choice jobs that are opening up elsewhere in the organization.

- *A peer* from another functional area of your organization. In organizations, knowledge is power, and the more you know about what is going on in other areas of the organization, the more effective you will be. Sharing information with colleagues is a necessary strategy in today's flat organizations.

- *A subordinate* who will level with you. From time to time, you need to know how you are regarded by the troops. If your people are restless or unhappy, they can find a hundred ways to make you look bad—and you'll never know.

- *A computer guru* to keep you up-to-date on the latest hardware and software. Information technology is changing so rapidly that you need to have informal access to an expert you can trust to steer you to new software and hardware that will make you more effective in your job, while warning you away from new information technology that has proven to be troublesome.

- *A former classmate.* Alumni often form close friendships that continue long after graduation. A special bond exists among alumni that can open doors at critical times in your career, such as when you are thinking about changing jobs.

Should You Invest in an MBA Degree?

The MBA is a management degree, and not everyone is interested in becoming a manager. For example, half the engineers who were surveyed plan to continue as technical specialists, so the cost and the time to earn an MBA degree would not be worth it to them. Similarly, physicians who have no interest in management would gain little from pursuing an MBA degree.

But if your goal is management, an MBA degree is indispensable, for two reasons:

1. It is an efficient way to gain many of the 10 Strategic Skills that our survey respondents found valuable for their personal and professional success.

2. It provides permanent certification that you are professionally qualified as a manager.

The most powerful endorsement for investing in an MBA degree comes from those who have already made this investment and have seen it pay off. When survey respondents holding an MBA degree were asked, if they had it to do over, would they still go for an MBA degree, 92 percent answered "yes"—an overwhelming level of customer satisfaction.

Economic Advantages of Earning an MBA

Although financial gain is not the only reason for pursuing an MBA, for many prospective students it is an important one. The total investment, including forgone salary, to earn an MBA in a two-year, full-time program can easily exceed $100,000. Is it worth it?

- Data from the survey showed that the median pay for men and women at age 30 who hold an MBA degree ($60,000) is twice that of those at age 30 who have only a typical undergraduate degree ($30,000).

- For survey respondents who graduated from the full-time MBA program, post-MBA starting pay was typically 50 to 70 percent—and in some cases 100 percent—above their pre-MBA pay.

- Furthermore, post-MBA pay grew rapidly, compounding at 10 to 20 per-cent per year during the first 5 years after graduation, much faster than the 5 per-cent raises that are common today.

A present value calculation of the financial return on the investment in a high-quality, full-time MBA degree program shows that, for most graduates, the degree easily pays for itself in the first 5 to 7 years after graduation.[5]

Quality-of-Life Advantages from Earning an MBA

In addition to the financial rewards for investing in an MBA degree, many of the survey respondents emphasized that they were able to draw on the knowledge and skills acquired in business school for many important decisions outside of their jobs, such as buying a house or managing their investments. Their MBA degrees also gave them a disciplined way of approaching the management of their careers, because many of the skills learned in business school—strategic planning, marketing, analytical skills—are directly applicable to the management of one's "company of one."

Furthermore, respondents reported that a major benefit of the MBA was the freedom it provided in pursuing a wide variety of career paths—from an investment banker earning more than $900,000 a year to a mother who was delighted to be able to return to the workforce after raising her children. Formerly employed by a major international accounting firm, she now serves as an accountant for her local church at $25,000—modest by MBA salary standards, but it's a job she loves.

Options for Earning an MBA Degree

There are three traditional options for earning an MBA degree, all of which are described in greater detail in the following chapter.

The two-year, full-time MBA degree is the program of choice for those who can afford to take time off to pursue an MBA. Many top schools require two to four years of prior work experience before entering their programs. The summer internship between the first and second years is particularly valuable to those who are switching careers from, say, engineering to investment banking.

Part-time MBA programs are best for those who currently have great jobs or who have family responsibilities that preclude taking two years off. Part-time programs take three to four years to complete. Data from the survey showed that post-MBA salaries are typically 30 percent higher than pre-MBA pay. The biggest problem faced by part-timers is getting their employers to recognize the value of their new skills following graduation.

Executive MBA programs are an excellent choice for those with 15 or more years of work experience. Students are normally on a fast career track with their companies and are usually in their late 30s. Classes meet all day once a week, usually on alternating Fridays and Saturdays to minimize time away from the job. Many physicians pursuing an MBA have found that the executive MBA is their best choice.

The One-Year MBA

On the horizon is a major innovation in graduate management education. In addition to traditional two-year, full-time MBA programs, a few top schools are introducing highly selective, full-time, one-year, accelerated MBA programs for exceptionally well-qualified students with substantial work experience. Similar to the top one-year European MBA programs at INSEAD and IMD, this innovation offers the saving of a year's time in starting one's career, and a large economic advantage—typically $90,000—by earning an extra year's pay at the higher post-MBA rate and by beginning to compound the rapid growth of this higher pay a year sooner.[6]

The one-year, accelerated MBA is an attractive option for physicians who are planning to enter management. Typical of the pioneering schools offering a top-quality, one-year, accelerated MBA program is the Roy E. Crummer Graduate School of Business at Rollins College in Winter Park, Florida. The Crummer School has made its program particularly attractive for physicians and other experienced health care professionals who would like to earn a high-quality MBA degree in the minimum possible time.

References and Footnotes

1. Lagnado, L. "Famed Cancer Center Gives in to Managed Care." *Wall Street Journal*, Oct. 25, 1996, p. B1.

2. Adapted from Yeaple, R. *The MBA Advantage: Why It Pays to Get an MBA.* Holbrook, Mass.: Adams Publishing., 1994, Chapter 2.

3. Yeaple, R. *The Success Principle.* New York, N.Y.: Macmillan, 1997.

4. In the sections that follow, space limitations allow only a brief overview of each of these strategic skills. For details on how to master these skills, see *The Success Principle*, Chapters 2-11.

5. For the details of this calculation, see *The Success Principle*, chapter 5.

6. For a more complete description of the new one-year MBA programs, see *The Success Principle*, pp. 250-5.

Chapter 2

What Physicians Can Expect from MBA Programs

Adele C. Foley, MA, MBA, and George W. Winter, MA

Physicians who report their activities in MBA programs are overwhelmingly positive about their newly acquired knowledge, their new methods of acquiring knowledge, and their new colleagues. Their expressions of interest in and support of management education in no way deprecate the value of their medical schooling and the competence of their colleagues and instructors; quite simply, they have discovered something new and useful that was not a part of their professional lives until they began exploring formally the strange, and perhaps exotic, world of business. They were learning to use knowledge that had not intruded on their relationships with patients and colleagues, to employ methods that in some ways seemed directly opposed to the scientific methods they had been taught, and to work with colleagues who cheerfully shared responsibility for work and results.

In fact, physicians contacted for this chapter were not merely pleased with their graduate business study; they expressed an almost youthful exuberance with what they had discovered and with the dimension that discovery had added to their professional and personal lives.

"Something Totally Different from What I Had Ever Studied:"

Generally, business knowledge is different from medical knowledge, but a number of physicians believe that some business issues and the knowledge required to deal with them clearly belong in medical education. Viewing the patient as customer attracted the interest of physicians studying marketing and operations management at both St. Joseph's University in Philadelphia and Minnesota's Carlson School of Management. They describe their studies much as Dr. Leonard B. Nelson, Co-Director of the Pediatric Ophthamology Department at Will's Eye Hospital in Philadelphia, compares his MBA emphasis on the customer at St. Joseph's with his medical studies at Harvard: "I was able to learn something totally different from what I had ever studied." Carlson School's Dr. Chris Alban, a full-time day program MBA student and a board-certified emergency physician, describes a similar experience in slightly different terms: "MBA studies introduce topics that the physician realizes should have been taught in medical school. For instance, focusing on the patient as customer and on patient service (as opposed to treatment) is absent from most medical school curricula, but heavily emphasized in MBA curricula."

Physicians also find marketing, budgeting, and investment courses valuable in their practices and in their personal financial activities. Some report having been formerly at the mercy of office managers or accountants when they had to make business decisions about their practices, departments, or hospitals. Graduate business study gave them the confidence to make independent judgments.

"I Keep Looking for the Multiple Choice."

Many favor what they call "non-quant" courses. Communication skills, human relations, strategic thinking, and leadership seem to fascinate these bright, competent scientists and healers. Physicians are as interested in the *approaches* of business study—to problem solving, decision making, and learning—as they are in the knowledge itself. Dr. Kenneth Veit, Dean of the Philadelphia College of Osteopathic Medicine (see Chapter 5), believes that medical education is "historically facts-oriented, with an alleged correct answer. Business education is more group-focused and process-oriented. The predominant linear thinking of medical school is replaced by a more conceptual and abstract process" in business education. Dr. Veit's feeling that "team courses and group-dynamic learning require a new patience that many physicians find uncomfortable" is echoed by Dr. Harry Manser, a physician in private practice in New Jersey, who puts the perception in slightly different terms: "In medical school, we were taught to be self-sufficient and independent, to work things out for ourselves and come to our own conclusions. Physicians do not want to give up control. The typical physician finds it hard to step down and share power. Business uses a method of thinking that is 180 degrees opposite the one we used when we were medical students." Graduate business schools, especially those with requirements that students spend at least three years in responsible work between their undergraduate and graduate programs, emphasize that students and professors learn from each other, that students share responsibility for learning.

Medical schools are beginning to adopt some of the approaches to learning that have been hallmarks of business schools for many years. Case studies, for instance, have been appearing in some medical school courses for the past several years. Carlson School's Dr. Alban believes that people currently in medical school may find graduate business study somewhat more compatible with their graduate medical programs than did their predecessors.

"Old Facades Began to Melt Away."

Nevertheless, one feature of graduate business programs that consistently pleases most physicians is not likely to appear in medical schools. The diversity of MBA student bodies is comparable to few other graduate professional schools. Most medical schools select students overwhelmingly from a pool of young high-achieving undergraduate students with "premedical" backgrounds primarily in the physical and theoretical sciences. Most MBA programs select students from a variety of backgrounds—English, history, political science, biological sciences, engineering, theater arts, music, business, philosophy, and economics—and from a broad spectrum of ages, predominantly from the mid-20s to the mid-40s but including people in their 50s and 60s. Also, because most U.S. business schools see the arena of commerce as international, many have developed liaisons with schools in other countries, and a large percentage of MBA enrollment in U.S. institutions is international and speaks English as a second language.

Dr. Craig Alan Winkel, Vice Chairman of OB/GYN and Head of the Reproductive Endocrine Division at Thomas Jefferson University Hospital in Philadelphia, states that his MBA classes were the first time that he "had been in a large group not composed of physicians, nurses, and scientists." Paul Edwards, a full-time Carlson MBA student who left medical school after two years to pursue a career in business, comments that the most pleasant surprise in the MBA program is "the variety of backgrounds of MBA students. You can learn so much from your fellow students."

The views of Dr. Winkel and Mr. Edwards represent those of most of the physicians interviewed for this chapter. During their MBA studies, many medical people developed friendships with their classmates from different backgrounds. As they worked with people in nonmedical fields, some discovered that their "old habits and facades began to melt away." They discovered that the world of medicine made heavy demands on their private lives and severely restricted their ability to socialize with people outside their profession. MBA studies opened up social and cultural possibilities that had never occurred to physicians in their demanding profession.

"All—And I Mean All of It—Has Been Very Interesting."

What physicians will learn in MBA programs varies somewhat by type of program (executive, part-time, full-time, or joint), but in all programs students can expect to learn the foundations and the core elements of business. Because these fundamentals are taught on the graduate level, professors cover the material more rapidly than one finds at the undergraduate level, and they expect students to learn much of the material outside of class through extensive reading assignments.

The MBA, like most professional and academic master's degrees, emphasizes breadth of knowledge, and most program courses assume that outlook. The heavy reading assignments characteristic of some programs reflect the intent in business courses to stress the wide-ranging knowledge that modern corporations expect in their managerial employees. Physicians, who are accustomed to in-depth examination of a smaller amount of material, experience some initial difficulty with this different view. Dr. Nelson illustrates the differences by relating how his Harvard Medical School classes would focus on one organ at a time and examine intensively all facets of its composition and function.

As discussed in the preceding chapter, foundation courses in MBA programs emphasize both breadth of knowledge and the relationship of seemingly different disciplines in the modern corporation:

- **Financial Accounting.** Principles of accounting and financial statements. The course will appeal to the logic and linear methods of the student of science but will cause some initial confusion because of its abstract concepts.

- **Statistics and Data Analysis.** Statistical method, interpretation of data, regression analysis, inferential procedures. "Old hat" to the physician whose premed program emphasized mathematics.

- **Behavioral Science/Organizational Behavior.** Theories governing individual, collective, and institutional behavior. The emphasis on diagnosis and on applying theory to organizations may appeal to the diagnostic inclinations of the physician.

- **Information Systems/Management.** Computers and how they can be used to manage and produce information. Because most medical students today are thoroughly familiar with computers, this course should be a natural and interesting expansion of that knowledge. However, physicians who have been out of medical school for five years or more may find themselves struggling in the first phases of the course. Many schools have prematriculation familiarization courses to help students get up-to-speed in computing.

- **Managerial Economics.** How markets work and how they are affected by events, incentives, political systems, and industrial structure. This study will be new to most medical people, but it is one of those courses that appeal to physicians, perhaps because of their newness.

- **Human Resources.** Theory and practice of managing people at work; hiring, developing, and compensating employees; motivation; job design; and labor issues. Another new concept for doctors. However, they find this course interesting because it deals with people issues in a way that departs substantially from doctor-patient relationships. In this course, physicians look at people in a different way from the view they have been accustomed to take.

Students round out their foundation courses with principles of finance, marketing, and operations, all of which have no counterparts in medical school or in most physicians' practices.

Today, MBA programs emphasize real-world relationships among basic elements of business as they merge two or more of these courses through team-teaching and interdisciplinary exercises. Viewing people as instruments of an economy, as employees of an organization, and as an element in profit or loss will confuse someone who looks at people as healthy or unhealthy organisms. Dr. Winkel, a spring 1997 graduate of St. Joseph's executive MBA program, describes some of these courses as a "transition away from the medical science of black and white to the gray areas of business." He comments that people who rely on clear decisive answers are often frustrated in business classes when someone answers a question, "It depends."

In full-time day and part-time evening MBA programs, students move on to concentrations and electives after they demonstrate mastery of basic studies. Concentration courses advance students' knowledge of a single business field so that they can establish themselves more credibly as experts in that field. However, students also take electives to broaden their knowledge of business and to gain credibility with their breadth of ability. In the following examples of concentration and elective courses, one can see a somewhat greater degree of specialization and advanced knowledge:

- Production and Inventory Management

- Managing Service Operations

- Psychology in Management

- International Financial Management

- Futures and Options Markets

Joint medical/MBA and law/MBA programs allow fewer concentration and elective courses because students' time in the programs must be split between management studies and medical or legal studies. Similarly, because of weekend scheduling constraints, most executive MBA curricula are characterized as "lock-step" programs, in which all students study the same subjects with no time flexibility for electives and concentrations.

Many MBA programs have "capstone" courses that students take in their last quarter or semester as evidence of their having mastered the theory and practice of business. Schools regard these courses as the means of "pulling it all together" so that students can experience a higher level of interdisciplinary problem-solving activity or bring about a synthesis of experience, knowledge, and theory. Live-case team consulting projects, leadership courses featuring a series of top-shelf CEO speakers, courses in business ethics requiring a paper extensively exploring a moral issue—all are examples of courses designated as "capstones."

"There Was an Absence of Hierarchy."

This comment by a physician well into his MBA studies suggests that how MBA students learn may trigger the biggest adjustment that physicians will make during their years in graduate business study. Some physicians felt that medical school was more rigorous than graduate business study, yet others described business study as more demanding. However, all physicians who provided information about their MBA experiences commented on two features of the approach to learning they discovered in their programs: the relative absence of authority and the shared responsibility for learning. These characteristics of the MBA classroom are in step with the tendency in contemporary organizations to "flatten" their organization charts and eliminate levels of hierarchy that narrowly define employee roles and breed the tendency toward bureaucracy.

Business schools are following suit and are eliminating or "scrambling" the old departmental concept of organization, sometimes called the "silo organization" because of its tendency toward isolation and vertical (in-depth) study. Because the MBA is a professional, not an academic, degree, business schools must meet the expectations of the business culture, which seeks employees with breadth of knowledge, networking skills, and the ability to communicate effectively across departments and specialties and with people of different cultures.

This transition may not be easy for physicians who are accustomed to hierarchical, authoritarian relationships. Most of the physicians who related their experiences described this feature of graduate business study as a problematic "surprise." They appeared glad to experience it, but hesitant in adapting to it. Dr. Winkel contends, "There is a hierarchy in medicine that you must respect. Physicians have spent their entire careers learning and understanding that hierarchy. That is not true of modern business culture."

Dr. Winkel adds that, as a result of the influence of authority and a pattern of vertical communication, many physicians "do not talk to each other" effectively. "That is why many physicians are not good negotiators," Winkel emphasizes. The desire of the business world for people with strong communication skills and the ability to build lateral relationships may cause adjustment problems for some kinds of physicians in MBA programs. Dr. Alban notes that medical generalists (e.g., internists, family practice physicians) tend to be more effective leaders of medical teams and coordinators of group efforts because they have more of a "big-picture" orientation than do specialists and surgeons. Although in the medical world successful surgical or specialty practice requires an intensely myopic view and an adherence to absolute authority in the operating room, success in the business world is more apt to come to someone with a broad democratic view, who can establish productive relationships with people in a number of different fields.

There is no question that surgeons and specialists, intelligent and competent as they are, can adapt their organizational concepts and communication styles to the needs of business; however, they should be prepared for a period of adjustment as they contemplate graduate business study.

The distillation of modern corporate culture has resulted in the team approach to study, a form of business school pedagogy that is first a cause of frustration and later a source of joy to the physician, who has no educational precedent for it. Dr. Nelson, enrolled part-time in St. Joseph's evening MBA program, states, "The group approach is definitely not done in medical school. You may discuss a patient in a group, but you are not into group projects." Dr. Manser, also part of the St. Joseph's evening program, admits that initially he found the concept of teams difficult: "It is not what you do as a physician, particularly in private practice."

Teams, however, are a fact of life in business, and they are now standard operating procedure in the MBA classroom. However, working with a team creates additional stress in scheduling and attending team meetings and in preparing one's own share of the work. Most physicians who have adjusted to this mode of study find both additional stress and welcome relief working with their team members. Team members share the work load and rotate leadership positions; they share their knowledge and responsibility for learning. Also, teamwork appears responsible for the benefit that doctors cite most often—working with people of different backgrounds and different approaches to problems. Doctors are discovering what business has known for many years: The more points of view that one can bring to a problem, the better the chance of solving it effectively. Teams will have a prominent place in international business and in the MBA classroom for many years to come.

The Four Basic Kinds of Learning Communities

The four predominant forms of MBA education have arisen from and adapted to student needs—time, money, and interest.

Academia's Weekend Warriors

Executive MBA (EMBA) programs enroll more physicians than other programs, perhaps more than all other programs combined. Normally meeting on alternate weekends or every weekend on alternate days (Fridays or Saturdays), these two-year programs offer a special style of study for people who cannot give up their jobs or practices and who work late in the afternoon or early evening with sufficient frequency to make part-time evening classes impractical.

Most EMBA students come from the world of commerce and industry and are sponsored by their employers, who pay for their tuition partially or wholly and allow them time away from work to attend classes, team meetings, and special activities. People who, in the minds of their employers, enjoy that level of confidence are generally bright students and responsible classroom colleagues. The experience of working together through heavy study assignments and strenuous problem-solving exercises develops durable friendships and desirable business relationships among students. Physicians in private practice, hospital administration, and other health care organizations become a part of these advantageous networks and form social ties to people outside medicine.

Dr. Veit, a graduate of Temple University's executive MBA program, cites as his most pleasant surprise his "fellow classmates, especially the non-health care types, who provided a pleasant break from doctors, nurses, *et al.*" He praises the special "bonding of people from many different backgrounds to achieve."

Physicians enrolled in EMBA studies enjoy the special treatment accorded to this select group of students. They find the maturity of their classroom colleagues particularly pleasing, and they find both their new knowledge and their new approach to knowledge refreshing.

EMBA course work is highly compressed, for programs must pack large amounts of learning activity into brief periods of instruction and disrupt minimally the vocational and personal lives of students. Because most students bring more than 10 years of responsible work experience to the classroom, instructors use a seminar style of exchange, relying heavily on the experiences of students for a large part of the course content. In order to engage the participation of students, manage the limited class time effectively, and see that sufficient knowledge is imparted and accessible to students, most EMBA directors hire their schools' most mature and productive professors to teach.

In most EMBA programs, learning generally takes three forms: (1) the on-campus or conference-center residency, (2) the regular and rhythmic Friday-Saturday schedule with an occasional Thursday thrown in, and (3) the one- to two-week international seminar abroad. This variable approach to study and learning helps to engage students' interest and anticipation and to prevent the compounding of boredom and end-of-the-week fatigue. Programs consist of about 15 to 18 months of classroom study; each degree program spans most of two academic years. Some schools suspend classes during the summer; others cease operation only during about 30 days of mid-summer.

In most programs, students carry the equivalent of 9-10 semester hours or 12-13 quarter hours of class work, and, with few exceptions, EMBA students take the same courses at the same time (called the "lock-step" schedule) as they progress toward the degree. Generally, courses have traditional titles (Financial Accounting, Information Technology Management, Operations Management), but some courses are specifically designed for the concerns of the EMBA student (Leadership Challenges, Ethics and the Legal Environment). Individual class periods run two to four hours and mix lecture, seminar give-and-take, and small-group discussion and problem solving. Guest lecturers on highly specialized topics are common throughout the curriculum. Most programs choose professors who are accomplished speakers as well as authorities in their disciplines.

With the limited time for class meetings, EMBA programs require that students "hit the deck running." Heavily laced with opportunities for camaraderie, most get under way with social events and orientation "residencies" (sometimes referred to as "boot camps") at conference centers in which students relearn or get up to speed in the basics of personal computers, finance, statistics/mathematics, and study skills. When formal classes start, students share a basic level of knowledge and can work together in teams productively.

In many programs, students form teams during their first residency and remain on those teams for the entire two years of study. During orientation, some programs expose students to teamwork theory and teach them techniques for making teamwork more effective and for improving their contributions to team efforts. Emphasis on teamwork is virtually universal in EMBA programs, because it mimics the way most organizations perform work and facilitates the continuation of study and completion of assignments during the students' one- to two-week absences from the classroom. (Teams meet to prepare assignments between classes.) Also, because teamwork promotes students' learning from one another, it is a major selling point of the executive MBA program.

International residencies, another major selling point, have come a long way since their early days, when they were called, derisively, "group vacations." Programs treat these study tours as serious and necessary professional development, because the overwhelming majority of EMBA students are American or represent American corporations. Accordingly students are required to study the language and cultures of the countries they are scheduled to visit during residencies. Studying and experiencing the business cultures of other nations has become a hallmark of credible graduate programs in today's international business environment. American physicians who have been trained in American universities and hospitals will find the international emphasis of contemporary MBA programs both interesting and pleasurable. During international residencies they are likely to meet with health care administrators as well as industrial and financial managers in host countries.

Although most extracurricular benefits accruing to MBA students (treated below in the section on full-time day programs) are found in the full-time day program,

EMBA students have the opportunity to share many of those programs. They are invited to enjoy speaker series; use the services of professional writing, speaking, and team effectiveness coaches; and pursue employment opportunities through career service centers. Through their classroom contacts with thoroughly experienced fellow students and talented instructors, they can acquire an informal kind of mentoring relationship that is not common to other MBA programs.

The Challenge of Functioning on the Edge of Being out of Control.

The Part-time Evening MBA Program, often called the "traditional" program because of its popularity a half-century ago among early MBA students, enrolls a considerable number of physicians whose schedules allow them an occasional weeknight clear of practice and on-call duty. Like the EMBA, part-time programs allow physicians to keep their practices and positions in other health care organizations as they make progress toward the MBA degree. Also, depending on the size of their medical work load and their personal responsibilities, they can take either a light or a heavy course load. Nevertheless, one doctor described the difficulty of maintaining his medical and hospital duties and studying for his MBA as "the challenge of functioning on the edge of being out of control."

Unlike in the EMBA program, part-time students can select courses from the same number and variety available to full-time day MBA students. They can choose concentrations in a variety of fields, and they can broaden their business knowledge with scores of elective courses. Minnesota's Carlson School of Management is typical of large universities in offering more than 90 advanced business courses to its part-time MBA students.

Part-time MBA programs are designed for working professionals. Typically the range in ages, vocations, backgrounds, and interests of students is extremely broad. Most courses are offered once a week in the evening, and some schools, such as St. Joseph's University, have extended their class schedules to Saturday mornings for the convenience of students who are finding themselves pressed by work and family responsibilities in the evenings. Also, part-time study allows students to balance their work, personal, and study responsibilities with the flexibility of assuming light or heavy course loads that match their obligations outside the university. Part-time MBA programs allow students up to six years to complete their degrees, although most students receive the degree after two to four years of study. Students in many part-time programs find additional flexibility in the credit given them for undergraduate preparation, work experience, and their ability to demonstrate a high level of competence in skills such as writing and speaking.

Part-time programs permit single and double concentrations in a variety of fields, including such standard subject areas as accounting, finance, information systems, and marketing. In addition, many schools offer specialization opportunities in health care management, medical services administration, or hospital administration. Physicians who wish to specialize in any subject area must, of course, satisfy foundation and core course requirements. The flexibility of the part-time MBA allows physicians to design programs that meet the demands of their practices or their positions in health care administration and that satisfy their special needs for additional knowledge and skill.

Part-time evening programs contain a number of the extracurricular features of full-time day and executive MBA programs. However, just as part-time study is not as intense as full-time study and because part-time students spend less time on campus, students encounter and enjoy these experiences less intensely than do full-time students. Nevertheless, much of the rich networking and social opportunity common to MBA study is present in the evening part-time program. Although the busy schedules of doctors allow them to spend relatively little time on campus, they find that they do have time to make friends with colleagues before, during, and after class, and the team method of study brings them into close relationships with fellow students as they collaborate to complete course work. Physicians, as graduate business students, are invited to a variety of university events, such as speaker series, receptions, and special networking opportunities at local clubs and restaurants.

Also, many part-time programs offer two- or three-week study tours to Europe, Central America, Asia, and Australia. These three-credit tours commonly include about eight business organizations, and graduate students have the chance to meet and discuss the culture and nature of business with their hosts. To prepare for the tours, students are expected to study the culture, businesses, history, and languages of the host nations and to present their findings to their colleagues who will accompany them. Similarly, after the tour, students are expected to present what they learned in lengthy papers. Students who travel together often form friendships and meet together socially for many years after the experience. Because experiences during the study tours are expected to meet the needs of students, physicians who enroll for the travel experience may expect to find opportunities to study systems of health care in other countries.

Part-time students at universities with career service centers and communication improvement programs can take advantage of these opportunities to improve their careers and abilities. For physicians who are considering different practice or administrative opportunities, career service centers can provide important services throughout a professional job search. Those who wish to improve their communication skills can find professional help with writing, oral presentations, interviewing skills, and conferences with patients.

You're Going to Do What?

The full-time day MBA program has become the most prestigious, or the "flagship," business program at most universities. The annual rankings of full-time MBA programs are generally considered to encapsulate the worth and the prestige of the entire business school. However, these programs enroll fewer physicians than other forms of MBA study because of the severe restrictions they impose on other kinds of activity. Most full-time day MBA programs consist of two, nine-month years of intensive synergistic learning. From September to May or June of both years, MBA students experience "total immersion" in a program of study and activity with colleagues from virtually every kind of background and from many nations and cultures.

Full-time is not for everyone. The experience is so intense and time-consuming that physicians with more than two or three years of practice after residency or internship should consider another approach; once a physician is heavily invested in a practice, full-time MBA study is probably out of the question. Because full-time programs will not permit physicians to spend more than 20 percent of their time practicing medicine, only those with insignificant ties to practice will be able to take on the burden of full-time study. Dr. Alban feels that doctors more than a year or two out of residency should take a different approach to the MBA: "They should consider an executive MBA or a part-time evening program. If you want to study full-time, you must be prepared to leave your practice. Even limiting medical practice to one day during a weekend is a moderate strain on a full-time student's schedule." Physicians in administrative or teaching positions may want to prepare for full-time study by acquiring their business foundation courses in part-time programs and then taking a year off or a sabbatical to finish their degrees in full-time programs.

The Accelerated Alternative

For physicians who have substantial business or administrative backgrounds or whose academic backgrounds include a number of business or economics courses, the accelerated or "advanced placement" (AP) MBA alternative is worth considering. After starting in a summer session, AP students gain their degrees after 12 months of study and graduate at the end of the following spring quarter or semester. Because AP students have most or all of their foundation courses, they can begin immediately taking concentration and elective courses. They integrate quickly with the students in the second year of their two-year program.

The Typical Program Commitment

The typical program that a physician may expect of full-time study consists of about 16 quarter credit-hours or 12 semester credit-hours of classroom study. For every credit hour, a student is expected to spend 2-3 hours per week in study (including class time). However, students report that their actual commitment to classroom and outside-of-class study and activities is actually double the guideline (4-6 hours for every credit hour). Team meetings, oral presentation practice, guest lectures, and special tutorials extend a full-time student's commitment to 60-80 hours per week. Carlson School's Mr. Edwards lightly refers to the outside-of-class work as "busy work" and recalls his first two years of medical school as devoid of such applied learning as oral presentations, team competitions, and collaborative writing assignments . "Medical school is entirely given to individual study—chiefly science and math—with no emphasis on collaboration and cooperative skills."

Most full-time programs consist of foundation courses, concentration courses, and electives. Most schools present fundamental business subjects in a way that displays their integration and interdependency in the modern corporation. Students in two-year programs commonly encounter foundation courses that integrate the fundamentals of statistics, accounting, human resources, organizational behavior, finance, marketing, and information systems, which sometimes are taught by interdisciplinary teams of faculty. In these courses, students demonstrate their integrative ability in business games, cases, competitions, and team oral presentations.

After 15-20 weeks of studying business fundamentals, most two-year full-time students enroll for courses in their chosen concentrations and in electives designed to "round out" their preparation. Students in the full-time or AP program, whose backgrounds already include most business fundamentals, can begin to work on concentrations and electives in their first quarter or semester of study.

Extracurricular Enrichment

In full-time day MBA programs, extracurricular activities rival curricular activities as learning opportunities. Mentoring programs, speaker series, consulting opportunities, employment-related activities, social activities, and special skills training claim the few hours still available in the calendar of MBA students. Nevertheless, whatever the strain on students' calendars, these activities are some of the most worthwhile experiences to be had in the full-time day program.

Mentoring
Many MBA programs assign students to a volunteer mentor from a nearby business community. Commonly representing executive or upper levels of management, mentors meet with their assigned students once or twice a month to discuss student interests, study programs, employment opportunities, and techniques of managing organizations. Students contact their mentors for personal and career advice and for answers to business questions. Periodically, all students and their mentors get together for cocktail or dinner socials followed by a speaker or panel presentation.

Speaker Series
Most full-time day programs sponsor series of speakers on business-related topics. Some speaker series constitute a credit-bearing course, such as a series of CEOs addressing requirements for organizational leadership, and students are required to research the speakers' organizations and relate the speakers' comments to specific features of, or developments in, their organizations. Also, business schools are particularly alert and have special funds set aside to pay for scholars, writers, and business professionals who will speak to students and faculty in classrooms or at special gatherings.

Consulting Opportunities
Because more and more MBA programs require that applicants for admission have three or more years of responsible work experience, the average MBA student can contribute sophisticated knowledge to classroom discussion and, in concert with other graduate students, help solve complex interdisciplinary problems encountered by organizations in local communities. Consequently, many business schools sponsor volunteer teams of MBA students who provide help free of charge to charities and not-for-profit organizations. Volunteer consulting can benefit substantially from the participation of physicians, because community clinics and special health programs are often in need of management assistance.

Some two-year full-time programs make team consulting and entrepreneurial start-up coaching a part of the second-year curriculum. The consulting experience gives the student approaching graduation an opportunity to work with two or three other students in solving a problem considered "major" by a business, government agency, or not-for-profit organization, all of whom pay a substantial fee to the school for the services of an MBA field consulting team. Because students are assigned to teams according to their backgrounds and interests, physicians can seek assignments in the health care field or venture with their team members into nonmedical business territories.

Employment-Related Activities
Perhaps the most anticipated and energy-charged service provided to all full-time MBA students is the "career services" activity. Career service centers provide

placement services, schedules and accommodation of corporate interviewers, resume books, libraries of corporate information, information sessions with prominent national and international companies, assistance in resume and "cover letter" preparation, and supervised practice in employment interviewing. These activities attract most students, and the career service centers are lively hubs of students seeking internships, jobs, and sophistication in the skills that people need to mount a successful employment search. Corporations that rely on MBA programs for strong job candidates schedule several days of interviews each year in school facilities and sponsor "information sessions"—cocktail parties with speakers—for students interested in the companies.

Social Activities

Because students in full-time day MBA programs study together, attend the same extracurricular programs, compete with each other, congregate in the same lounges and study areas, and cooperate to solve problems and complete assignments, they tend to bond and socialize together. Social activities for MBA students range from end-of-the-week beer and snacks in the lounge to formal dinners and dances. Golf tournaments, intramural athletics, barbecues, house parties, and pub crawls take place throughout the academic year. Because of the rigors of the program and the need to encourage students of different backgrounds, skills, and cultures to work together, it is common for schools to encourage and underwrite part of the cost of social activities. Formal meetings and speakers are often followed by food and refreshments and opportunities to congregate with guests, faculty, and fellow students.

Skills Training

Training in special software, oral presentation, writing, team effectiveness, intercultural negotiation, and other skills necessary for success in business take up a relatively small, but significant, portion of students' schedules. Often considered "soft skills," these subjects are some of the most durable and important to the careers of people in business. Universally, physicians react well to "soft skills" training, especially to working with others and sharing responsibility for outcomes. Some respondents pointed to the reluctance of doctors to give up control and to share responsibility with colleagues; others said that medical school trained them to be self-sufficient and independent, to work things out for themselves. However, many physicians commented that, once they became accustomed to working in groups, they felt more relaxed and enjoyed learning from others and relying upon their judgment.

To Prevent the Need for Catching Up

DO/MBA programs are one of a number of cooperative programs (the law-school version, JD/MBA, is another) that couple graduate work in two professions and award degrees in both. Originating at the Philadelphia College of Osteopathic Medicine, the DO/MBA program stems from a growing awareness of the importance of business in medicine and of the need to equip many physicians with strong managerial skills before they find themselves in positions that require them. The growing number of managerial positions in the health care industry derive from continuing changes in the way medical services are organized, delivered, and paid for. Many organizations actively recruit doctors for these positions.

Dr. Robert Cuzzolino, Associate Dean of the Philadelphia College of Osteopathic Medicine (PCOM), recognizes "the need for physicians to acquire the MBA as part of their medical training, for the very practice environment that makes this training so valuable today nearly negates the opportunity for young physicians to achieve it." Dr. Cuzzolino is concerned that "the demands of an active practice" will prevent many competent physicians from taking advantage of "expanded opportunities in a field that is now governed by traditions of corporate organization, marketing, and business."

More than seven years ago, PCOM joined with St. Joseph's University in a cooperative effort to provide management education for students in osteopathic medicine. So far, the DO/MBA program has had a 100 percent retention rate, and, in the past two years, the number of students in the program has doubled.

Future physician executives study business concurrently with their second and third years of undergraduate medical education. The students divide their time equally between medical education during the day and graduate business education in the evening. The course of study consists of 12 MBA courses, each student taking two courses a semester (summer, fall, and spring) while taking half their second-year medical studies in each of these two years. In May of the second year, they are awarded the MBA degree, and they take their board examinations. The students then complete the remaining two years of medical training and are able to schedule their rotation cycles without conflicts.

A Flexible Advantage for Physicians

The MBA carries both tangible and intangible advantages for new physicians. The degree gives them access to several fields, including utilization review and quality assurance, and to positions of leadership in managed care or medical provider organizations. Students who do not see themselves with a future in medical management nevertheless see the MBA as a credential that identifies them as special candidates for clinical appointments and as formidable competitors for residencies. The MBA identifies the candidate as a physician with an additional dimension of leadership ability and with both analytical and interpersonal skills. Also, knowledge and skill that physicians acquire on the path to the MBA enable them to rely less on business advisors and consultants in handling their practices.

Postscript: an Advantage to the Institution and to Other Medical Providers

As an outgrowth of the joint DO/MBA program, St. Joseph's University expanded its program by offering specialization in health and medical services administration to all practicing physicians and people in the health care industry. The medical management courses have become popular with area physicians, who find the late afternoon, evening, and Saturday schedule of courses convenient. The University has developed a group of specialized courses (e.g., Accounting and Finance for Health Care Management, Health Care Economics, and Health Care Systems) that are restricted to students with backgrounds in the health services field. In the final semester of their MBA studies, medical students, physicians, and other health care professionals take a special capstone course, entitled Strategic Management in Health Care Organizations, that covers formulation and implementation of organizational strategy and business policy processes in the health care industry.

Conclusion

Doctors who feel that they would benefit from advanced business education and an MBA degree will find that U.S. higher education has provided ample opportunities for them. However, despite the availability and convenience of graduate business programs, physicians should prepare carefully to take advantage of this opportunity to study. First of all, they will have to prepare for the Graduate Management Admission Test (GMAT), which is required by most schools of business. More important, they will have to prepare their families for their frequent and sometimes lengthy absences for class attendance, team meetings, and study, and they will have to arrange their office schedules to accommodate this new time-consuming activity.

Drs. Alban and Veit recommend that physicians have specific objectives for taking up graduate business study. Both feel that the rewards of MBA study are substantial, but that, in order to reap those rewards, doctors must invest a great deal of time and energy. Some doctors consider medical school more rigorous, while others consider graduate business study more demanding. All agree, however, that the MBA work load will have a major effect on a physician's work and family.

Also, doctors will need "to melt their facades" and prepare to share power and knowledge. They should prepare themselves to keep an open mind and not prejudge their courses, fellow students, and professors. Doctors should be prepared to find some courses and knowledge that seem "fuzzy" (as one physician put it), but if they accept the responsibility of studying the material, it may prove valuable at a later stage of their study. They will find fellow students who know more about subjects than they do, and they will find others who communicate more effectively. Initially, some physicians may find that hard to accept. Finally, they will encounter instructors with a wide range of "stylistic differences"—some tightly structured and authoritarian and some, seemingly unstructured, who will give students latitude to shape their own learning. The advice of colleagues who have been in the graduate business classroom is not to be put off by style and to concentrate on the substance behind the method.

Despite the newness and the strangeness of some parts of the business curriculum and culture, physicians soon find themselves acquiring the language and accepting the culture of business. They perform well and uniformly are glad they took up the new challenge. Dr. Craig Winkel sums up the response of his colleagues: "Wish I had done it ten years earlier."

Chapter 3

A Survey of MD/MBAs: Is This the Future for You?

by Mary Frances Lyons, MD

L et me preface this chapter with some caveats so that there is no confusion, as otherwise this would read as a commercial for an MBA degree.

Caveat 1: MD/MBAs are a minority of the total number of physician executives today, and that situation is not likely to change any time soon.

Caveat 2: Health care organizations do not, in my experience, hire physician executives solely (or even largely) on the basis of the MBA degree. It is merely one of many factors.

Caveat 3: I'm not advocating the MBA for all MDs. Organizations still rely on "chemistry" in making their executive selections. An MBA may help, but experience and credibility count more.

My work as an executive search consultant takes me daily into the health care job marketplace. I wanted to know what MD/MBA individuals have to say about the value and importance of the degree in their own careers. So, I went straight to the source with a simple survey, and the results are reported in this chapter.It's not an over-statement to say that, just a few years ago, physicians who had a little management experience and an affable manner were considered well-prepared for careers as physician executives. Those days are gone, but a quick overview of the marketplace for physician executives suggests that the meager "qualifications" of a few years ago have been replaced by equally unrealistic expectations. Today, it is assumed (wrongly) that every candidate will be a super-doc with an MBA degree from a prestigious university. (Affability and management experience still count, too.)

We have come to expect that clients today will ask for individuals with MBAs as candidates when we are engaged in physician executive searches. The clients may not always hire MD/MBA candidates, but they expect to see physicians with that degree in the short list of candidates for their senior positions. (Heard about some recent consumer research on vending machines? Snickers® candy bars were the most popular vending-machine snack food, but people surveyed said they wanted to see more healthy snacks. So the companies added healthy snack choices to the selections. Know what happened? Sales of Snickers® went up, and everyone was frustrated because the Snickers® bars sold out faster. They finally figured it out:

Consumers had it right. They wanted to see the healthier snacks; they did not, however, want to buy them. I sense some important parallels here, how about you?)

There is a gap between the idealized, MBA-toting MD and his or her real-world counterparts who are among the thousands daily performing well, meeting the challenges of their work as physician executives in hospitals, systems, integrated delivery networks, managed care entities, insurance companies, pharmaceutical firms, and many other locations. Some of them have MBAs; as of now, most do not.

Why did some already highly educated and accomplished MDs choose to pursue an arduous degree-seeking path to achieve an MBA? And what do they think its impact has been on their careers? Do they receive financial help from their employers? Do they feel the MBA has contributed to their success as physician executives? And how has it effected their professional lives? Would they advise others to take this course?

These are interesting questions, and to explore them I conducted the nationwide survey of MD/MBAs mentioned previously. A random sampling of 75 physician executives who have already completed an MBA degree was sent the questionnaire and invited to participate; 30 individuals (for a respectable response rate of 40 percent) responded. I'm grateful to all who took the time to share information and insights with me and their fellow physician executives.

When Did They Start/Complete Their MBA Degrees?

On average, respondents began working on their MBAs in 1988 and completed degree work in 1990. Thus, the respondents are not fresh out of school. Rather, they are a group of physician executives who have worked at least several years since they acquired degrees. Their perceptions about the impact of degrees on their careers and the usefulness of the degrees would seem to be more valuable as a result. The earliest MBA completion reported was 1984; the latest was 1996.

How Long Did Degree Completion Require?

The table on page 31 shows that the actual time needed to complete the degrees varied, although the majority completed a two-year program. This relative speed suggests a certain urgency, since most respondents completed their MBA degrees without stringing it out over a number of years, as they might have done. In all, more than three in four completed their degrees in one or two years.

Those who have delayed making a decision to pursue an MBA because they have concerns about how long it might take to complete one should note the relatively brief time commitment reported by respondents. The clear message: An MBA is doable for an MD, even by those who remain employed as they complete classes, reading, and other requirements. It is clearly difficult, but not impossible.

What Type of Academic Programs Did They Utilize?

The majority (75 percent) of the physician executives responding said they had participated in executive MBA programs. These programs are usually designed for individuals

Time to Complete an MBA Degree

Number of Years	Percentage of Respondents
1 year	14%
2 years	64
3 years	7
4 years	11
5 years	4

who are working full time; often, the coursework and assignments are geared to the specific career goals of participants, who are already in mid- or senior-level roles. The remaining 25 percent completed degrees in " typical business school programs." In either case, these programs frequently require some period of working experience prior to entry.

Not surprisingly, none of the respondents said they had received their MBAs in "a physician-specific MBA program." These programs have become more visible only in the past few years, and this survey population, on average, completed their MBA degrees in 1990. My own view is that physician-specific programs may be too narrow in scope and may not provide a full range of perspectives and viewpoints.

Richard Streck, MD, MBA, is currently Vice President, Medical Affairs, at Akron General Medical Center. Reflecting on the value of his MBA training, which was completed in an executive MBA program, he said: "Like many others, I saw the writing on the wall. If physicians were to have significant influence in health care decision making, we would need to learn to speak the language of business. My MBA school experience was fascinating; business executives really do think differently from physicians, and altruism is foreign to their bottom-line mindset. But I also learned to work in groups and to see that the collective decisions we make are always better than the best individual decisions. Today, when I use my business school background to communicate with physicians in our organization, I may still see myself as a physician, but I know that my colleagues see me as an administrator."

What Was Your Primary Reason for Completing an MBA Program?

Respondents offered a variety of reasons for obtaining MBA degrees. In rank order of importance (the number of times mentioned), the reasons are:

- Business knowledge and skills (most mentions).

- Credibility as an administrator.

- Knowledge to function effectively on the job.

- Named/selected for administration.

- Interest in management.

- Career advancement.

- Survival in the era of managed care (least mentions).

These responses are fairly predictable and offered no surprises. In fact, I interview MD/MBAs every day who give these as their reasons for seeking the degree. Those who are considering embarking on an MBA program should compare their own motivations with these and talk with a mentor about the results. If one of them isn't your primary reason, think again about moving forward with the idea. It's similar to embarking on a weight-loss program; to be successful, you have to do it for yourself and for no one else.

Did Employer Pay Some or All of Cost of Your MBA Degree Program?

For 68 percent of respondents, their employers paid no part of the cost of their MBA degrees. Twenty-nine percent said their employers paid part of the cost, while, for 3 percent, the employer paid ALL of the cost. A few respondents suggested an "in-kind" contribution, mentioning that their employers allowed them to take time off for classes and research work involved in their degree programs.

Increasingly, we note that physician executive candidates include career development (particularly tuition reimbursement for management degree programs) as one of their key negotiating points with hiring hospital and health system organizations, and financial or compensatory time support for MBAs is appearing as a condition of employment in the contract requests of those already in physician executive positions. As we learned in a 1996 survey of CEOs about their physician executives, CEOs are generally interested in providing educational assistance to this newest addition to the senior management ranks. One desperate CEO remarked: "Would pay for courses, a degree, seminars, etc.—any of the above—if they would just do it!"

It seems clear that physician executives should sound out their own CEOs on this matter. Federal income tax laws on tuition reimbursement have changed often in the past few years, and this is an additional factor to be considered by all parties.

What Has Been Impact of MBA on Your Career as a Physician Executive?

Eighty-nine percent of respondents said the impact of the MBA on their careers has been positive; 4 percent said there had been no impact, and 7 percent said they did not know the impact. (In the latter category, individuals said they had completed it too recently to have made an assessment.) No one claimed a negative career impact resulting from an MBA.

The statements made by our respondents are an overwhelming endorsement of the pursuit of MBAs in enhancing their careers. From hundreds of interviews throughout the country over a period of years, I can attest that those with MBA backgrounds generally are more enlightened in their thinking than physicians in general may be. While the material one studies for an MD degree consists of facts, a body of knowledge, the MBA material involves principles, ways of seeing problems and appreciating points of view that may be different from one's own. I think of the MBA degree experience as "the gift that keeps on giving."

Daniel Whitlock, MD, MBA, Vice President of Medical Affairs at St. Cloud Hospital, St. Cloud, Minnesota, commented on how his business training has affected his life and work: "As a pediatrician treating respirator-dependent children, I saw that their medical progress was affected by public and private business decisions as well. I entered an MBA program to learn how to speak the language of business and to ensure that the care was delivered. Today, as a 'boundary person' between hospital administration and physicians, I design linkages such that the financial information in a profit and loss statement is reflected in the care that is delivered. My executive role is another way of delivering patient care; when I certify quality or design systems, I am seeing that people get the help they need. It's very satisfying work."

Some typical write-in comments on the impact of the MBA degree on careers include:

- I am no longer practicing medicine; I am now a stockbroker.

- It meant I could leave practice five years ago.

- It has been valuable for my advancement, for credibility, and for day-to-day information required in my position.

- It made me more confident and gave me a broader perspective on the position of health care in the overall economy of the United States.

- It is nice to have but not critical or even necessary.

- It gave me tools and perspective that are not usually available to classically trained MDs.

- I gained business credibility.

- It allowed me access to the sales/marketing side of the pharmaceutical industry.

- It has given me more insight into finance and human resources management issues.

- It has given me new ways of thinking and new ways to approach problems.

- It has opened doors not previously available.

- It changed my career.

As executive search consultants, we often hear from physicians who have completed their management degrees but who lack any meaningful management experience. These individuals sometimes expect to be selected at once for top jobs in huge, complex organizations, but that is unrealistic. Just because a physician achieves an MBA or another management degree, he or she is not instantly endowed with management expertise. Would the new graduate from medical school be employed to perform complex surgeries? Not until he or she has been further trained. Similarly, a new MBA also requires seasoning and experience before the most senior positions are attainable.

Young physicians graduating from medical school may feel ready to take on any challenge, and newly hatched MD/MBAs may have more confidence than experience; both will need to pay their dues before they can rise to senior roles. Some recognize this; some do not.

Would You Advise Others to Embark on an MBA Program?

Most respondents (82 percent) said they would advise others to embark on an MBA degree program, while only 4 percent said they would not (half-humorously, the comment was made: " I don't want the field to become too crowded"). Interestingly, 14 percent said that the advice would depend on how deep was the interest and how pressing the need. Morris A. Flaum, MD, MBA, chairman of medicine, St. Joseph Hospital, Ann Arbor, Michigan, says: "Formal management education has given me a number of invaluable tools to which physicians are not usually exposed in their training, such as strategy development and implementation, cost accounting, finance, and organizational behavior. In completing the MBA program, I also gained insight into the processes by which decisions are made in the nonmedical setting."

The message from respondents on whether they would advise others to seek MBA degrees seems to be that it was worth it to them, although, of course, it guarantees nothing. Their write-in comments included:

- You should be a full-time administrator [to pursue an MBA].

- If you do not pursue it, you might otherwise expect to work for nonMD/MBAs.

- When the influence of HMOs diminishes in the coming years, physician executives will have an advantage [with an MBA].

- It's a comprehensive learning experience.

- It will open your eyes and broaden your knowledge.

- It offers physicians new career potential.

- It depends on what you already know and where you want to go.

- Without an MBA, you can't really understand the business/administrative viewpoint.

- It gives you the business skills you need to succeed today.

- Medicine needs clinically trained physician executives to offset the strictly businessman approach to health care.

- It helps you to understand general business, especially cost-accounting.

- Be sure it is a high-quality program with 100 percent on-site instruction, and be sure that you have a career goal.

- Only if it is applicable to a real job, and not a fantasy that he/she will become a super-CEO.

Would You Do It Again [Seek an MBA] Today?

Almost the entire respondent group (96 percent) agreed that they would do it again today. This is a far higher percentage than I expected to see, given that an MBA is costly and time-consuming and cannot be assumed to lead to a new career path. Only one individual said he would not do it again, citing family responsibilities and saying it was too time-consuming. A respondent commented jokingly (one assumes): "It's cheaper than a mistress (and safer)." Other write-in comments included:

- The MBA experience provided new information and stimulation.

- It was enjoyable to be back in school.

- It broadened my vision.

- I have greater credibility and information I need.

- I am better able to deal with business executives.

- It's proof that you can retrain your brain after age 50.

That last comment is particularly telling, as it follows my own thinking on this matter. Only a few years ago, I was recommending that physicians under age 45 who were interested in changing careers consider pursuing an MBA. Today, I recommend that physicians of any age look into the business degree opportunities that may be available to them, precisely because it is an enriching experience that can provide intellectual stimulation and exciting new working options.

Conclusion

While I am glad to know that the sampling of MBA-holding MDs I surveyed are so enthusiastic about the degree, I want to make it clear that I am not a strong advocate of the MBA per se. It seems to be working for a number of people, but it is hardly a universal solution to the question of how to move into management ranks. All the degrees in the world will not qualify an individual for most key jobs. It is the combination of the degree and the right kinds and varieties of experience that can be so powerful. The best career credential is experience, but, given the apparently insatiable appetite for learning of most physicians, it is not surprising that they are pursuing MBA degrees in increasing numbers.

What should you do? You should think it over, long and hard, before you make any irrevocable moves. Take a course or two and see how it goes. Talk to people who have MBAs and hear their points of view. Talk to your boss and ask for an assessment of the MBA's potential impact on you and your career path. If you listen to anecdotal material by the physicians who responded to this survey, you could easily believe that the MBA is essential. Deciding whether to "go for it" could be your first—and most far-reaching—management choice. How you decide may be less important than the fact that you gave it serious consideration.

Chapter 4

From Bedside to Business School: A Personal Odyssey

by Arthur Lazarus, MD, MBA

Why would any self-respecting physician want to go to business school? The question has many answers, depending on whom among the nation's 16,345 physician executives[1] you talk to.

For many physicians, an MBA is a gateway to a fast-track health care management path. Having chosen such a path for myself, I knew that business training and an MBA degree would become increasingly important for my curriculum vitae. Classified ads for physician executive positions frequently state a preference for an MBA degree. A medical degree alone may be insufficient to climb the corporate health care ladder.

If nothing else, graduate business training teaches physicians the language of business. Before I entered business school, I had never heard terms such as "economies of scale" and "value creation." I thought "providers" furnished goods and services, not clinical care. I thought "first mover advantage" was a concept in rehabilitation medicine rather than marketing. I laughed when I first heard the term "loose bricks" in a strategy course. But then what did I know about the medical lexicon before I entered medical school?

Identification with the Aggressor

I never planned to go to business school. In fact, I never was very interested in the "art of the deal" or in fraternizing with business people. I was interested, however, in psychology and management theory, subjects that attracted me to the psychiatric profession. I figured I could further my training by going to business school and concentrating on the qualitative aspects of management. Peter Robinson, author of *Snapshots From Hell: The Making of an MBA*, describes people like me as "poets": students in business school who lack a business background, are interested in the softer side of business, and appear to be "numbers blind." It's not that quantitative courses in finance and accounting are beyond my reach; I just dislike working with numbers. To this day, my wife balances our checkbook.

Business people are a thorn in the side of physicians. When I worked for a utilization review organization, a physician remarked that I had identified with the aggressor. Like most physicians, he was outraged by the intrusion of corporate values into medical practice. He was concerned that I would be corrupted by "Big Business" and become a slave to the bottom line.

Another physician labeled me a double agent. He figured that, by working for a utilization review organization, I could improve quality from the inside. Perhaps as an insider I could focus the attention of senior management on quality concerns rather than cost containment. I could be the superego for the company!

In reality, it came down to the fact that I needed to go to business school to obtain a foundation I never had in college or medical school. Ultimately, my thirst for additional knowledge guided me back to the classroom. Perhaps going to business school was my midlife crisis, although I was hoping my midlife crisis would have been a little more flamboyant than this.

The Executive MBA Solution

I was uncertain how to obtain an MBA degree quickly and without interrupting my career. The solution came to me while browsing an educational supplement to the *Philadelphia Inquirer*, where several colleges advertised "executive" MBA programs.

There were four programs within 10 miles of my home. Two programs were not accredited. The third school was high-priced and high-powered, an Ivy League college with tuition in excess of $70,000 (now $80,000). The fourth school, affiliated with my medical school alma mater, had a reputation for high-quality, affordable education. Tuition for the two-year program was $27,500; my employer covered about 30 percent of the cost. Additional features of the program included:

- Twenty-one-month course of study.

- Classes given on alternating Fridays and Saturdays.

- Broad-based program in general business.

- Strong emphasis on faculty interaction and peer group learning.

- Courses taught by instructors with business savvy.

Typical of many executive MBA programs, class size was small (23 students). The average age was 37, and about one-quarter of the students were female. Students had an average of 11 years' work experience prior to matriculating. One-third of my classmates had previous graduate degrees representing diverse backgrounds in engineering, arts and sciences, and technical areas. Our class was divided nearly equally between accountants, engineers, and health care professionals. Students were mid-level or senior-level managers.

The program fee included all instructional costs, course materials (books, case studies, and readings), required software, program-sponsored events, and meals and refreshment breaks. The fee did not include the purchase of a laptop computer and participation in an international seminar. Some executive MBA programs do, however, include study tours abroad as part of the tuition package.

Table 1. Executive MBA Curriculum

First Year

Fall
Financial Accounting
Business Statistics
Organizational Dynamics

Spring
Management Science
Microeconomics
Strategic Management

Summer
Macroeconomics
Information Technology

Second Year

Fall
Managerial Accounting
Operations Management
Business Ethics

Spring
Finance
Marketing
Human Resources Management

Summer
International Business
Strategy Formulation and Administration (Capstone)

The executive MBA curriculum is predominantly lockstep—i.e., courses are prescribed and taught in sequential order, as shown in table 1, page 39. Study groups are an integral part of the learning experience and also teach students how to work in teams. Members of each class begin the program at the same point, move through most courses together, and usually complete requirements for graduation as a group. A few executive MBA programs offer electives, but the majority do not provide specialization or offer a concentration in health care management.

Executive MBA. programs are highly intensive, and completing them is certainly not a "gimme." We lost two students after the first year. One student, a physician, left for personal reasons. The other student returned to her native France when her husband was transferred. Business school, perhaps more than medical school, is unforgiving if you have a personal crisis. There is no "retention committee." I changed jobs midway through the program, but I would not recommend taking on that added stress unless absolutely necessary.

Undertaking an executive MBA program requires fortitude. I was physically and mentally challenged. In dealing with the ups and downs of students, the executive director of my program realized that business school took on a life of its own. She said there is a "life cycle" that students go through over the two-year course (see

Table 2. Executive MBA Student Life Cycle*

Stage One: Orientation through First Semester

Symptoms: Anxiety, norms created, high energy
                   Underlying issues of self-worth activated
                   Concern about time demands on family, work, self
- Feeling moderately eager with high expectations.
- Feeling some anxiety. (Where do I fit? What is expected of me?)
- Testing the situation and central figures.
- Depending on authority and hierarchy.

Stage Two: Dissatisfaction

- Finding a discrepancy between hopes and reality.
- Feeling frustrated, unable to get things done.
- Feeling incompetent and confused.
- Reacting negatively toward leaders and members.
- Competing for power and/or attention.

Stage Three: Resolution

- Gradually increasing satisfaction.
- Resolving discrepancies between expectations and reality and between conflicts and misunderstandings.
- Developing harmony, trust, support, respect, self-esteem, and confidence. Giving more feedback.
- Sharing responsibility and control.

Stage Four: Production

- Feeling excited about team activities.
- Working collaboratively and interdependently.
- Showing high confidence in accomplishing tasks.
- Sharing leadership. Feeling positive about successes.
- Performing at high levels.

Stage Five: Termination

- Feeling concern and possible stress about the break-up of teams.
- Feeling sad or gratified.
- Decreasing or increasing activity and morale.

Stage Six: Transition

- Life without business school.
- Separation from school and loss of support group.
- Career change: Use it or lose it.
- Feelings of tremendous pride and accomplishment.

Courtesy of Marie L. Zecca, Director, Executive MBA Program, Temple University School of Business and Management, Philadelphia, Pennsylvania.

table 2, page 40). Business school has a significant impact on students' families as well.

Apart from class time, expect to spend 15 to 20 hours per week on assignments. There are mid-term, final, and other exams, plus class projects and papers, both individual and group. I found that the key to completing the program was having a well-functioning, cohesive study group and allotting sufficient time to do the work.

There are more than 100 executive MBA programs to choose from nationally. Make sure your school is accredited by the American Assembly of Collegiate Schools of Business. Although you will probably be limited by geography, a few executive MBA programs offer long-distance learning via computers and teleconferencing. Because of the special nature of the executive MBA curriculum, all course credits must be taken within the program. Previous graduate work in business school may enhance your performance, but the credits are not transferable. Likewise, executive MBA credits are not transferable to other types of MBA programs.

The Financial Factor

The real advantage of an executive MBA program is that you can continue to work full time while in school. Nevertheless, business school is an expensive proposition. Most physicians who have been out of medical school more than 10 years will experience "sticker shock" at the price of tuition and wonder whether the cost will be justified by future earnings. No hard data exist, but, according to *Medical Economics*, physicians with management degrees tend to earn about 7 percent more than those without a degree.[3] A physician executive compensation report conducted in 1997 by the Physician Executive Management Center, Tampa, Florida, found that the median total compensation for full-time senior medical managers in hospitals was $186,000; in managed care organizations, $187,000; and in group practices, $181,500.[4] Physician executive compensation tends to rise faster than the rate of inflation. Moreover, newly hired physician executives typically earn 12 percent more than their nonmedical CEO colleagues.[5]

Another type of cost-benefit analysis was published in the *New England Journal of Medicine*.[6] Using standard financial techniques to determine the return on educational investment over a working lifetime for five groups of professionals—primary care physicians, specialist physicians, dentists, attorneys, and graduates of business schools—researchers found a superior financial return on the educational investment when students chose a career in business compared with primary care practice. The results of the analysis indicated that an investment in professional business education leads to a path of financial reward.

Ronald N. Yeaple, Executive Professor of Business Administration at the University of Rochester, New York, conducted an in-depth study of business schools in the United States (see Chapter 1). He concluded that there was indeed an "MBA advantage," at least for nonphysicians attending top business schools. The MBA advantage has two components: a two-year increase in pay that occurs upon graduation and a post-MBA five-year fast track salary growth. The economic value of the MBA degree is higher for more research-intensive schools. Executive MBA programs appear to be an especially good investment, considering that there is virtually no opportunity cost to attend these programs.

The Business Personality

Once in business school, I evaluated whether the business field was right for me. Admittedly, this put the cart before the horse, but the results of the evaluation did confirm the goodness of the fit.

The Strong Interest Inventory, a measure of career interests, suggested that my career goals in business were compatible with my basic interests in medical service and science, teaching, and writing. These interests, in turn, correspond to activities such as managing, instructing, and analyzing and processing data. According to the Strong Interest Inventory, individuals with my interests are particularly suited for careers in business and psychology. Inasmuch as I am a psychiatrist, assignment to the latter category is not too surprising!

The Myers-Briggs Type Indicator (MBTI), a psychological assessment, showed that my personality closely matched the profile of a typical businessperson. My personality was characterized as introverted (I), sensing (S), thinking (T), and judging (J). The profile of the quintessential businessperson is the same, except that he or she tends to be extraverted (E) rather than introverted. Thus, my decision to enter business school appeared to be validated by two widely used screening instruments. The fact that the same person who aspired to go to medical school and become a psychiatrist is the one that decided to become an executive speaks to the changing nature of one's interests over time.

Most physicians are introverted, intuitive (N), feeling (F), and perceiving (P), especially psychiatrists, who tend to score the highest of all physicians on the intuition scale. I developed intuitive skills through years of medical training and treating patients in psychotherapy. These skills remain the only real vestige of my career in psychiatry. My "STJ" distinguishes me from most other physicians, yet my "I" distinguishes me from nonphysician managers. Essentially, my MBTI profile reflects a mixture of medical and business attributes, which may explain why I do not identify totally with either administrators or physicians.

Understanding differences in personality types has very important implications for improving relations between physicians and nonphysician managers. By recognizing differences at unseen psychological levels, one can more readily appreciate the roles and functions of health care managers. This is no small feat, because relations between physicians and administrators have been fraught with conflict for a long time. Also, awareness of psychological differences between physicians and managers may improve communication and working relationships. As health care becomes more managed, only a strong framework of trust and understanding will narrow the rift between physicians and administrators.

Practicing Versus Managing

Trying to maintain a private practice in conjunction with a full-time administrative job is probably more challenging than trying to reconcile some of the fundamental differences between physicians and administrators. Indeed, I have come to believe that the two endeavors are essentially incompatible.

Full-time medical management requires the same intensity and commitment to work as does patient care. Management cannot be viewed as a hobby or take a back seat to practicing. Similarly, a busy practitioner cannot afford to interrupt his or her schedule to respond to frequent administrative dicta and deadlines. Conceptually, I believe it makes more sense to focus on skills training for medical managers and concentrate on practice essentials for clinicians. The more serious one is about a career in administration, leaving practice to devote full time to management, the more important it is to have an MBA.

One of my business professors commented, "Management is not for amateurs." His comment was prompted by an incident in which two supervisors mismanaged the termination of an auto plant worker. The disgruntled employee returned to the factory and gunned down his supervisors. When the case was discussed in class, I was planning to lay off three physicians in a hospital downsizing initiative. The terminations were painful, but, thanks to my professor, I'm still alive!

MBA Cynics

Skeptics can't imagine blending medicine and business or replacing a clinical career with a nonclinical one. Prominent among the doubtful are family members of physician executives, the lay public, and medical organizations.

I remember when the American Medical Association (AMA) launched an advertising campaign and asked, "Would you rather trust your life to an MD or an MBA?" Recently, the following question appeared in an advertisement for a large health care organization in *Time*: "When someone's hurt, nobody ever yells, 'Is there a hospital administrator in the house?'" These type of questions bother me, because they pander to a stereotype that casts physicians as clinicians without administrative capabilities. By magnifying the differences between physicians and nonphysician managers, comments such as these widen an ideological gap that assumes that one person cannot fulfill both roles.

Soon after I graduated from business school, an academic advisor told me that an MD was "overkill." "You didn't need to go to medical school," she quipped, "you simply could have gotten your MBA in health care administration after you finished college." I proceeded to explain that administrative decisions in medicine are being made in a vacuum, that one person who understood both the clinical and fiscal realities of health care was better than two. But I'm afraid my reasoning was lost on her. In her opinion, medically untrained individuals sitting before computers with bottom-line-oriented algorithms were just as effective.

In addition, the Dilbert factor is at work. Scott Adams's popular cartoon character and many television sitcoms portray managers as morons unworthy of respect. Nowadays, much of the workforce wants nothing to do with management, a major shift from just a decade ago when employees strived for the golden ring. They cite the stress of handling bosses and subordinates, ending up in the middle. According to the *Wall Street Journal*, management phobia is running rampant in corporate America.[7]

Many people think physician executives should continue practicing to subsidize their salary and to maintain credibility among other physicians. One MD/MBA said that he dropped the MBA after his name so he wouldn't be perceived by his peers as having joined the "suits." But who are the peers of dual degree holders? Other physicians? Nonphysician managers? The answer, of course, is both, because, ultimately, physician executives lead a double existence.

Conclusion

Reflecting on his experience in business school, Peter Robinson felt that, for all its trials, the education was worth it—not as a straight and easy road to riches but rather to gain an appreciation of the brains, talent, and sheer creativity required in business.[2] Robinson, a former speech writer for President Reagan and now a fellow at the Hoover Institution, left the White House to attend Stanford Business School. He mused that business school did not deliver his classmates into paradise, but it did equip them to lead interesting lives here below. My own experience has been no different.

Physicians who are interested in managing at an executive level cannot go wrong by having an MBA. There are career opportunities in many fields, for example, in academia, consulting, and the pharmaceutical industry, to name a few. The chapters that follow survey a wide range of career pathways in medical management. More than ever, physicians with MBAs are filling those slots.

References

1. *Physician Characteristics and Distribution in the U.S. 1996/97 Edition.* Chicago, Ill.: American Medical Association, 1997, p. 13.
2. Robinson, P. *Snapshots From Hell: The Making of an MBA.* New York, N.Y.: Warner Books, 1994.
3. Mangan, D. "Lured by the Promise of a New Career? Read This First." *Medical Economics* 70(22):159-69, Nov. 22, 1993.
4. Kirschman, D., and Grenbenschikoff, J. *Physician Executive Compensation Report: A 1997 Survey of Physician Leadership.* Tampa, Fla.: Physician Executive Management Center, 1997.
5. Lauer, C. "Publisher's Note: Dear Physician." *Modern Physician* 1(3):9, July 1997.
6. Weeks, W., and others. "A Comparison of the Educational Costs and Incomes of Physicians and other Professionals." *New England Journal of Medicine* 330(18):1280-6, May 5, 1994.
7. Schellhardt, T. "Up the Ladder." *Wall Street Journal,* April 4, 1997, pp. A1,A4.

Section II
Career Pathways in
Medical Management

Chapter 5

Medical School Dean

by Kenneth J. Veit, DO, MBA

The role of the Dean of a Medical School varies from institution to institution. A common denominator is leadership and direction of and accountability for the academic program producing future physicians. An important aspect of this role is the many interactions with various operational units that accomplish the program's objectives. MBA education can be applied to these interactions. Specifics of the encounters can be difficult to quantify and define. The best analogy is perhaps a multi-tasking computer running multiple applications with MBA training running quietly in the background. The MBA skills constantly function in the background. When the occasion calls, this database of knowledge moves to the foreground. Perhaps "a day in the life" can add a sense of reality to the Dean's job and help better evaluate the utility of this additional training.

Any Day of Almost Any Week in Any Academic Calendar Year

After attendance at intern and resident hospital morning report and after a second cup of coffee, a day progresses in the following typical manner.

8:45 A.M. Meeting with the Health Care Centers
All medical schools, in various degrees, are responsible for clinical service delivery. Top medical educational institutions must strive to excel in education, research, and service. Very few schools excel in all three modalities, with most schools giving priority status to one or two. The elements receiving the highest priorities are either strategically selected or chosen by default. Each component functions as a business entity and therefore requires constant evaluation and monitoring. The component that perhaps drives today's academic centers farthest from their historic comfort zone is service delivery. Rapid change in service delivery today is making academic programs reassess their traditional norms. Academic medical centers with medical schools now merge and acquire hospitals and practices; at the same time, other medical schools sell or partner equity positions in these various units.

The issue on the table today is the ambulatory care component of the college. The discussion revolves around responding to the dual challenge of opening a new center and understanding the impact of complete capitation of medical assistance patients. This patient population comprises 85 percent of the current patients in the centers. This population, long neglected by private sector medicine, historically depended on educational training programs and hospitals to fill the gaps. Clinical services were not always delivered with unselfish institutional motives. Care of the indigent has always interacted with medical education. The impact of managed care on this population has brought the potential of new revenue. With this new revenue comes new competition in an arena that was for the most part noncompetitive.

Without getting into details, today's discussion revolves around marketing issues for the new site and around reimbursement concerns. The finance department would like doctors to expand hours, see more patients, and expand the capitation list. The doctors respond with concerns about teaching responsibility and the need to have higher personal compensation if their role is converting from pure academic to bottom line productivity.

Skills necessary to participate in the discussion run the gamut of financial insights into basic business tools, especially concerning the cost of the new site and the expected rate of return of a significant capital investment. The discussion also includes complex negotiation skills with both the finance department and physicians. Strategic planning issues are never far from the discussion. Core questions are addressed, such as "who are we and what is the business?" This theme continues throughout the discussion.

9:30 A.M. Meeting with New Clinical Chair
A new chair is in the process of completing the transition from employment with a private group to employment with the school. The issue at hand is the need to effectively communicate the new job. The job is a teaching and administrative position, a change from the familiar clinician role. The new chair desires clinical work. In the eyes of the institution, this is a secondary issue. The cost of clinical activity is high, especially with significant new clinical space and added personnel. The discussion involves a point of view that shared clinical space could provide the clinical activity desired without the added cost structure.

Discussions must adapt to the people involved. A discussion with a physician of a certain age and background cannot contain "MBA-type" language. The language is likely unknown and could indeed hurt the communication process. Discussions with the financial department, planning department, or board of trustees require a different set of strategies and skills. Although business and administrative skills are most helpful in this meeting, care must be given to be doctor first and administrator second in this particular interaction. Course work in communication skills from the MBA program continues to be very useful. Communication skills and experience from physician and patient relationships also translate well into many different arenas.

10:00 A.M. Meeting with Student Who Wishes to Withdraw from School
A student expresses the need to leave school because of family problems. After a time, the discussion has covered the implications of this decision for both parties, but the student still wishes to withdraw. The student decides to take a leave of absence for one year and to reevaluate the situation a year from now. A quick call to the admission director and student affairs office gives the assurance that the student's predicament could not have been prevented or influenced. The financial aid office is instructed to initiate the new status for this student and to counsel the student in loan and scholarship review.

The MBA thought process perhaps is not totally relevant in this scenario, except for the need to coordinate and communicate throughout the administration. The need to constantly reevaluate the outcome of the educational process is becoming increasingly critical.

10:30 A.M. Meeting with Web Site Development Team
Thanks to new technology, all institutions of higher learning are now being promoted in many new ways. Web technology and the current Internet did not exist in 1989 upon completion of the executive MBA program. One driving aspect of gaining MBA education was the personal desire to gain computer literacy. Perhaps the fear of a technology moving faster and the fear of being left behind drove the need for further education. Since 1989, technology has moved at speeds unimaginable just a few years earlier. However, because of core knowledge gained in 1989, the meeting progresses in a state of mutual communication. The MBA curriculum provided insights for this meeting and others that relate to new technology issues. The education also helps in the developing field of medical informatics, especially in relationship to medical education. In the work force and with the student body, e-mail and Internet access is not optional but routinely expected.

Today's meeting moves from technical possibilities to the site's structure and function. People at the table include the "techies" (and what institution can live without them), the Director of MIS, the Director of Marketing, and the Assistant Dean of Admission. A strategy develops to improve and enhance the Web Page.

This is a discussion that would not have occurred a few years ago. Dealing with change is now a constant in all industries. Managing change requires adequate tools, whether it is knowledge of new technology or of organizational behavior.

11:30 A.M. Conference Call with National Professional Organization
In any administrative position, one must deal with both the internal environment and the external environment. This particular conference call has to do with the planning of a retreat that involves reviewing the planning process and the strategic direction for the osteopathic college's national organization. All administrative positions have a political overtone. This is certainly true of a Dean's position. The ability to interact with the many different constituent groups improved with the executive MBA training, especially the informal curriculum. A group of successful mid-level professional people used the two years of sitting together in the classroom to become familiar with one another's work and personalities. Students participate in multiple group projects, gaining knowledge of one another's working environment. This interaction led to an increase in respect for different careers and different values of the group.

12:00 Noon Lunch with Prospective Students
An enjoyable part of the day is the occasional opportunity to sit with students before their medical school interviews. During these exchanges, one can best see the future in the eyes of these young people. Fear of medicine's change is not their concern. These prospective students want the opportunity to participate, and they dress for the occasion and act nervous as they wait their turns.

The lunch turns low key when we say that this event has nothing to do with the admission process. We discuss medicine, the school, and the unique culture and history of the osteopathic profession. "MBA 101" rarely enters the discussion, except for the occasional student's asking about the five-year dual degree (DO/MBA) program. This seems to be an increasingly popular option: to gain medical and business degrees in five years. For these students, the role of physician administrator becomes a part of their dream of achievement in medicine.

1:00 P.M. Graduate Medical Education Meeting

There is no better place in academic medicine to examine business concerns than in graduate medical education (GME). Not well known to the general public and perhaps to most students are the business and financial aspects of graduate medical education, otherwise known as internship and residency training. This training occurs after a primary medical degree is received. Graduate medical education training, subsidized over the past 30 some years by Medicare payments, remains critical for completion of the physician's formal education. Medicare payments for this education go directly to the teaching hospital of record. This payment is for the added cost of education and is a financial subsidy that contributes economic benefit to the hospital. This allowance has been a target of Medicare budget-cutters. The dollar amount on a national basis can vary dramatically, from $40,000 per resident to $150,000+ per resident. To society at large, the annual cost of this program runs to approximately $7.5 billion.

The college has a unique business concern with GME because of a slightly different model that has developed over the past five years. Because the college does not own a hospital, medical education, including internship and residency, function with affiliation agreements. The cost per intern and resident remains a college cost, with a negotiated agreement for payment from participating hospitals. The hospitals, in turn, use this "invoice" to receive Medicare educational cost payments.

The strategic challenge is to provide enough GME opportunities in high-quality teaching hospitals with negotiated agreements for payments that cover the absolute number of residents obligated. This is a very tricky business at best. It requires every aspect of MBA education, including financial analysis and forecasting skills (if not crystal ball reading). The meeting is just a prelude to calculation of college costs and sharing of this number with affiliation partners. A large part of the meeting is spent in reworking the agreement to reflect the concerns of the college.

This brings up another aspect of MBA curriculum, business law. Business law is just one aspect of the overall influence the legal profession holds in our society. The need to interact with the legal community on many issues stresses the need for mutual respect and some fundamental knowledge. Most law firms work "on the clock." Involving these experts in relevant issues is not only a critical legal concern but a budgetary concern.

2:00 P.M. Meeting with Director of Human Resources

Human resources departments present two critical issues today. The first discussion involves a case of alleged harassment by a faculty member of his research assistant. This complaint surfaced only after termination of the complaining individual. Discussion occurs over human resources policy and the need to follow-up carefully with everyone involved in the case.

The second issue concerns the decision to change the fringe benefit policy for prescription drugs for faculty. The change would have an impact on students unless the medical insurance company could provide this benefit within the current package and cost structure. The need to remain competitive in fringe benefits with the work force is critical as competition for the best employees accelerates.

The human resources course in MBA education is perhaps one of the most useful. On the surface, it might seem rather "soft" compared to accounting and financial courses. However, with the constant need to interact with the work force, whether faculty or staff, it remains one of the most relevant MBA courses. The meeting ends abruptly with a call from the clinic.

2:45 P.M. Emergency Patient Call
Often discussed by many physician executives is the role of their clinical activity. Does one attempt to remain an active clinician? This is not an easy decision. The credibility one has with the "white coats" remains with the physician executive as long as he or she is perceived as one of the group. Seeing patients and interacting with peers on the ward and in the clinic provides a framework that remains an administrative advantage. Leaving that arena means separating from much of the physician identity, knowledge base, and peer group. However, in a critical administrative position, the luxury of clinical practice can remain elusive and perhaps unfair to the patients. Clinical activity, even to a nominal degree, requires another level of commitment and support structure. This commitment is well worth the effort. Having current knowledge of the practicing environment, the frustrations, and the concerns of front-line clinicians can help immensely in the "board room." This advantage comes with a price. It likely will come down to an individual decision that is based on both self-motivation and the environment of the workplace.

The call from the clinic is from a patient with 15 years' experience with the organization. Concern centers on a recent change in his prescription and some mild side effects. The patient, once reassured, commits to an appointment at the next weekly session in the clinic. Any patients electing to continue with care must be aware of the limitation of availability and know the strict guidelines of back-up support. Patients must accept the limitations or accept alternative providers. A physician manager with a good back-up system can continue seeing patients and gains a sense of professional balance.

3:00 P.M. Meeting with Executive Group—Called by the President
A Medical School Dean is accountable to many parties. Access to the top of the administrative structure occurs with high expectations. Today's discussion revolves around two major topics. The first item is preparation for the board of trustee's meeting in two weeks and presentation of next year's budget. The budget needs fine-tuning one last time. The meeting is led by the chief financial officer.

The second order of business is to reassess the impact of new ownership of one of the major affiliated teaching hospitals. With the health care delivery system moving so fast with mergers and consolidations, the challenge remains to meet change with strategic discussion and flexibility in meeting mutual needs. A meeting time with the new owners, confirmed for the following week, concludes the meeting.

The executive MBA curriculum revolved significantly around the impact of change. How can one make change work for an institution? How does one effectively cope, deal, survive, and benefit in changing times? The health care arena is certainly feeling the full force of this "tornado" and perhaps following in the path of other industries, such as banking and retail businesses.

4:30 P.M. Meeting with the Student Council

Of the many constituent groups with which the dean relates, the student body is perhaps one of the most important. Time spent with this constituent group makes the job enjoyable. The issue on the table tonight is the role of the student ethics committee. The committee deals with issues of student behavior. The concern is the commitment by the dean's office to support this agenda. With assurances given, the second order of business is the student assistance program, which attempts to provide assistance and guidance to students on issues ranging from stress-related problems to potential addictive behavior and substance abuse. The need to work closely with the administration on these issues is critical for both the concerned individual and the institution's legal responsibility.

The administrative challenge in this activity is to function as the students' cheerleader and coach. Ultimately, the value of self-governance remains only as long as it remains self-governing. Allowing students, faculty, and staff the privilege and luxury to pursue challenges, supporting both successes and failures, can be most helpful to larger institutional concerns. Perhaps these concepts developed obliquely in the MBA managerial accounting class, a class that concentrated more on managing than accounting. As an executive, your ultimate job is to delegate and not necessarily "do." Your job depends on others, and effective delegation is critical for success. If this type of delegation is difficult, a top management position should be reconsidered.

Final Thoughts

The MBA degree remains an added value for a medical school dean. It provides a set of skills that is rarely directly applicable but that at the same time is constantly being used indirectly in various formats.

The personal decision to obtain MBA education came about with a slowly developing interest in administration. Certainly, for a young medical graduate, an administrative job was not part of any career direction. Preliminary interest in the need for more formal management education occurred during a three-year experience as a family physician in a very rural area. As a young National Health Service Corps physician practicing in a small town, needed skills exceeded the typical medical school curriculum. As the town physician, I found the need to interact with the community in many capacities. Serving on health-related committees, designing and building a new clinic, and advising on community needs became part of the routine expectations of the "town doc." In the academic world, many discussions ended with budget and business concerns, with a language base that was both strange and unknown.

The college offered to support participation in an executive MBA training program that met every other Friday and Saturday. It provided an opportunity to grow in a different discipline toward a knowledge base that that was both intense and challenging. The interaction and bonding that occurred with a group of fellow professionals, thrown together to tackle the classroom again, resulted in the most pleasant and rewarding surprise in the two-year experience.

Can a dean's job performance improve with an MBA degree? Academic deans with business training are still very much a minority. The individual dean's role can vary, depending on the culture and expectations of the institution. Does MBA training help in the day-to-day activity of a dean? Certainly for a dean with involvement in multiple activities, as the above typical day indicates, MBA training is always "running." The decision to attend an MBA executive training program was an excellent investment. The relevancy of all topics in the MBA training met many diverse needs. The program, unfortunately, did lack development in one very important business skill. The program failed miserably to help a pathetic golf game. This programmatic shortcoming was overshadowed by an excellent executive MBA training program that provided many critical skills, attitudes, and knowledge useful for this medical school dean.

Chapter 6

Health Care Consultant

by Spencer Borden IV, MD, MBA

The Origin of Change

The world of medicine started to spin out of professional control in 1982. The problem was that few physicians noticed.

At the time, I felt secure and content. I had fulfilled my career aspirations and was coasting, relishing my accomplishments. I was Radiologist-in-Chief at Children's Hospital of Philadelphia (CHOP), a 335-bed premiere pediatric hospital located on the grounds of the University of Pennsylvania. CHOP was highly regarded and was ranked in the top three children's hospitals by *U.S. News and World Report* for many years. All full-time staff held academic appointments in the Clinical Educator or Tenure Tracks of the University.

At age 35, I was recruited by CHOP and the University to rehabilitate the Radiology Department, which had fallen into disrepair after the departure of the previous Radiologist-in-Chief seven years earlier. My relocation to Philadelphia and acceptance of the position was conditional on full acceptance of my multimillion-dollar development plan for the subsequent five years, which I presented to the Hospital and the University in 1978. Much later, I discovered this was the first long-range plan of any type in existence at CHOP.

By 1982, my plan for the Radiology Department was completed. I had instituted three new imaging technologies: nuclear medicine, computed tomography (CT), and ultrasound. The radiologist staff increased from three to nine, total personnel from 31 to 143, and budget from $3 to $10 million per year. The training mission increased from three to 12 residents per year from nine regional training programs. A new pediatric radiology fellowship program, begun in 1978, expanded to two fellows per year and the fellowship term from one to two years. In 1982, the Department was a success and I was relaxing.

Symptoms of Change

During 1982, newspapers and popular health care journals were chronicling a new development: falling hospital admission rates and shortening lengths of hospital stay. Not just a regional phenomenon, these changes were occurring nationwide.

All the writers and pundits attributed these seismic events to the upcoming earthquake of hospital financing for Medicare patients by the Health Care Financing Administration (HCFA). As of July 1, 1983, HCFA would no longer pay hospitals their submitted charges based on a cost-plus formula, but would start a new payment system using fixed-sum payment rates for admissions, based on the diagnosis-related group (DRG) of the Medicare patient. Afraid of losing large amounts of money on each Medicare admission, hospitals encouraged their medical staffs to use fewer admissions and shorter stays for all patients. In short, hospitals were in training to operate in the post-DRG era.

This explanation was short, clear, appealing, and wrong. It missed the major point: DRGs were a symptom of something far more important, a dramatic power shift in health care. For more than one hundred years, hospitals and physicians had defined their services (admissions, office visits, physical examinations, etc.) and defined the charges affixed to these services. They routinely sent such charges to patients and, later, to payers. This payment method validated professional control of the health care delivery system. Up to 1982, no one had ever challenged that payment system.

If a payer redefines what constitutes a specific service and reconstructs how payment for that service is accomplished, it has assumed de facto control of the provider of the service. Providers will operate to maximize their economic returns under the new financial and behavioral incentives. The behavior of hospitals and their medical staffs in 1982 validates this conclusion. The use of DRGs for hospital payment proved that HCFA assumed total control of hospital behaviors for Medicare admissions. Clearly, once hospitals lost control of their payment methodology to external parties, physicians would be the next logical targets. However, few physicians understood their peril.

Recognizing these realities in 1982, my choices were clear. I could remain in my tenured position and wait for the tidal wave of disempowerment of physicians to engulf me at some time in the future. Or I could try to get ahead of the change process and affiliate with organizations likely to shape and control the future delivery of health care services. The former choice was familiar, comfortable, and troublesome only in the indistinct future. The latter choice was novel, uncomfortable, without a clear road map to pursue, and not at all certain of success. I chose the latter, but I did not know how to begin.

Barriers to Change

Practicing physicians are strongly acculturated during medical school, and that medical world view is reinforced during internship, residency, and fellowship training. I was taught that the only worthy endeavors of physicians were the famous legs of the three-legged stool: patient care, teaching, and research. Science was preferred over administration; money would follow good clinical practice for patients;

and people who were honestly trying to deliver good clinical care would naturally work together.

My experience in academic medicine taught me the Byzantine realities of high-power academic politics. The overall game is zero-sum; if you and your department succeed, someone else's will lose. Everybody wants to build an empire. The chips are clear: money, people, and space. Relative power is easily recognized by these criteria. Real friendship is uncommon among competing power brokers. Secrets inevitably leak, spreading at the speed of light through the internal grapevine.

My role as Radiologist-in-Chief had proved the value of understanding the role of management. Leadership required vision, commitment, endless communication, and understanding of the value of people with diverse backgrounds. My leadership efforts, though successful, were seat-of-the-pants management. I chose to build on my experiences in management. By this choice, I consciously abandoned a role of advancing the science in my discipline, pediatric radiology. I had no role model or road map, but I had to begin somewhere.

Breakout

Luckily for me, the University of Pennsylvania contained a full complement of graduate schools, including its School of Business Administration, the Wharton School. The Leonard Davis Institute of Health Policy in the Wharton School is nationally recognized for excellence in research in applied health science and health policy research. My next door neighbor, Dr. William Kissick, was a cofounder of the Institute and a big fan of management training for physicians. He encouraged me to apply for admission to the Wharton Executive MBA (WEMBA) Program, which met every other Friday and Saturday for two years, plus five full weeks of on-campus classroom work.

My consideration of business school drew stark and stereotypical responses. My friends in hospital management, accounting, and health care law thought it would be a fine opportunity. My physician colleagues thought it would be selling out, an abandonment of the medical profession, and would position me as a money-grubbing businessman. They were polite, but very blunt, in their criticism.

With trepidation, I applied to WEMBA for admission in 1984. My application was not helped by my GMAT scores, which, I was told, were those of a recent liberal arts major. Despite this, I was accepted.

WEMBA

The WEMBA program was tough, but fun. The first two weeks were crazy; more reading than could be done in one year, learning the names and habits of new classmates, and finding out what classes met where. Intentionally, it was boot camp for the new students. My class, the tenth at WEMBA (WEMBA X to the School), was 44 people, mostly midlevel managers who were looking to expand their careers within their own companies. I was one of two physicians. Many students had backgrounds in technical disciplines: engineering, physics, and chemistry. A few ran their own companies; others started their own companies in school and later.

Our class was empowered by one force: the knowledge base of our fellow students. We had experienced experts in everything. We constantly challenged the faculty with personal experiences. Most case studies would be picked to pieces by a classmate who was an expert in that industry niche. Study groups were formed and thrived. My study group of five gradually grew to 11, meeting every Monday night for the entire two years to dissect cases, review old exams and solve problems. Some students were discussion leaders, some niche contributors, and one could solve any problem with graphical analysis. Due to my dyslexia, I took voluminous classroom notes as my principal source of learning. Once discovered, this archive served classmates who liked to read more than attend class. I felt my decision to get an MBA had been ratified. I loved business school; I could run anything.

In retrospect, I made a fortunate choice to get an MBA. An MBA is the only graduate degree that expands the breadth of opportunities for the degree holder, allowing one to apply for new positions in one's industry or to consider lateral moves to a new industry. In my opinion, every other advanced degree (PhD, MHA, etc.) focuses one on a smaller range of endeavor by requiring greater in-depth knowledge.

The Transition

In late 1985, convinced of the correctness of my decision to expand my career horizons, I resigned my chair and faculty position, effective on the installment of my successor. Later, I came to understand that this decision was only possible because of my personal comfort with change and uncertainty and of my self-confidence. Other people, more risk-averse, would not have resigned their tenured faculty positions.

I finished WEMBA in May 1986 and received my MBA in June. The University and CHOP succeeded in selecting and relocating my successor in 1987. Now, in my second year after WEMBA, I was free to consider new possibilities. The options were numerous: hospitals, physician groups, industry, insurance, government, pharmaceuticals, and consulting. What niche was ahead of the power shift curve? What organizations were at the cutting edge? Where to begin?

At the time, I concluded that power rested with payers, given the example of HCFA and DRGs. I was recruited to Aetna Insurance Company in Hartford, Connecticut to start a medical technology assessment unit. The premise was clear and exciting: health care should be purchased, not just paid for, and those technologies that were effective should be covered. Those technologies that were not proven to be effective should not be covered for payment. After six months of research and personal interviews with national leaders of technology assessment, I submitted a modest proposal to establish an in-house medical technology unit staffed by six people. The proposal was turned down, because the employer who originally requested its formation had ceased to ask for it. At the time, Aetna considered itself a payer, not a purchaser, and felt that it could not interfere with the practice of medicine. (Years later, Aetna established just such a technology assessment unit, ably led by Dr. William McGivney). I was reassigned to review medical records and supervise nurse utilization review programs in five claims offices in the Midwest, a frustrating exercise. I resigned from Aetna after 15 months of employment.

In hindsight, this experience was not entirely a waste of time. I learned the operations and mindset of a large payer and had the opportunity to meet knowledgeable people around the country, many of whom are long-time friends.

The Management of Quality

In 1989, Dr. Alan Brewster and Charles Jacobs recruited me to join the company they founded, MediQual Systems, Inc., in Westborough, Massachusetts. MediQual had developed a software tool, MedisGroups, to measure severity-adjusted clinical outcomes (morbidity and mortality) of hospital admissions. The product had been selected as the measurement tool to measure the performance of all hospitals in the State by the Pennsylvania Health Care Cost Containment Council. During my employment, a similar initiative began for all hospitals in both Iowa and Colorado. As Medical Director of the Database Services Division, I became engrossed in the roll-out of statewide quality measurement initiatives, including education of and consulting to employers, health care coalitions, and state data-reporting agencies on the uses and limits of clinical quality measurements.

Alan Brewster introduced me to the topic of his passion: statistical quality control of health care. Statistical quality control, championed by Dr. W. Edwards Deming, involves systematic measurement of process variation in the formulation and delivery of both products and services. Managers must know the details and performance characteristics of the processes they oversee and the variations, waste, and comparative outcomes of the resulting goods offered to the market. Alan forcefully argued that statistical quality control of health care delivery must replace inspection quality control, the technique I had seen employed at Aetna. Understanding that quality could be accurately measured, that results could be publicized, and that managers could be held accountable for quality results has fundamentally changed how I have viewed the health care system ever since.

At MediQual, I became a good public speaker on issues of quality measurement, clinical outcomes, and public accountability, giving more than 100 invited presentations in four years. My sales and marketing experience allowed me to work with 45 business coalitions on health around the country. The pull-through marketing strategy of selling the need for hospital quality measurement software to the coalition and employer marketplace showed me the value of a consultative sales strategy. Our sales cycle was two years of high-energy collaboration, but the resulting hospital sales usually covered all hospitals in the region. We had success in Tampa and Orlando, Florida; Houston, Texas; Denver, Colorado; and Kalamazoo, Michigan.

MediQual experienced a dip in operating revenue during 1993. After two rounds of layoffs, my Division was eliminated in November 1993, and I was laid off. It was a huge blessing in disguise.

This time I had a clear picture of where I wanted to go. I had accumulated experience in academic medicine, management of physicians, payer management of employee benefits, quality and outcomes measurement, public speaking, and sales and marketing. My weakness was in consulting, which I had learned by the seat of my pants in my various positions. So, I needed consulting training and experience to round out my skills.

Watson Wyatt Worldwide

Chance favors the prepared mind. In mid-1993, I had the opportunity to meet Dr. William Mayer, who had just joined Kellogg in Battle Creek, Michigan, as Corporate Medical Director, and Dr. Roger Taylor, who joined PacifiCare in Cypress, California, as Chief Medical Officer. Both had left the Washington, D.C., office of the Wyatt Company (which later merged with Watsons of England to become Watson Wyatt Worldwide). So, thinking Wyatt may be short of physician consultants, I placed a call to Jim Braun, the National Health Care Practice Leader, whom I had met at our mutual client, ALCOA, in Pittsburgh, Pennsylvania. Candidly, I asked Jim how many physicians Wyatt had left, and his answer was none. That led to a dialogue, serial interviews, and my recruitment as Senior Medical Consultant for the Wyatt Company, located in the Boston, Massachusetts, office.

Like most of the major employee benefits consulting companies, Wyatt had a corporate headquarters (Washington, D.C.), various geographic regions, and many field offices across the country. The consulting staff consisted largely of actuaries and employee benefits specialists. The health care consulting practice focused on employers, but it was a growing practice with about 100 consultants scattered in Wyatt offices across the country. As I learned more about Wyatt, some important lessons became clear:

- Each Wyatt Office has a powerful office manager, responsible for his or her own revenues, costs, and profits. Office managers are in the majority on the Wyatt Board of Directors. In theory, each office and each practice in that office should be profitable. Corporate cross-subsidization of individual offices should be minimized. That meant that local projects should be performed by local consultants to keep revenues in local offices.

- Large, nationally based clients, such as General Motors and IBM, were managed out of corporate headquarters in Washington, D.C. The Washington office of Wyatt was well staffed, with more than 250 consultants, and was highly profitable.

- How scarce resources, such as physician consultants, were to be shared within Wyatt was never made clear. As consultants in remote Wyatt offices got to know me and my skills, I received more requests to do client presentations and to participate in projects in their regions. My time was cross-charged to the other offices, a negative incentive to use my consulting services. For two years, I was the only physician consultant in the company, so there was no alternative physician resource for remote offices to use.

- The life-style of a busy consultant is hectic. The compensation is very handsome, with excellent benefits, but there is little vacation time. Vacations reduce the hours available for billing. The travel schedule is intense. Many weeks, I traveled for all five days; at a minimum, I was on the road for three days a week. This life-style is grueling for the consultant, but even harder for one's spouse and children. The travel requirements may have been part of the reason Drs. Mayer and Taylor chose to leave Wyatt for more stable positions.

- Very few consultants in Wyatt were true colleagues, in that they understood the health care delivery system or had personal experience in delivering health care. At my arrival, there were four nurses scattered around the country; at my departure, there were fewer nurses and two new physician consultants, one the new Health Care Practice Leader.

- I had no colleagues in Wyatt who understood health care quality and outcome data and measurements the way I did. The only data sources were claims and enrollment data from employer clients, and Wyatt performed basic cost and utilization measures on these data tapes. Sophisticated clinical quality measures were not possible, and there was no facility to measure the performance of individual physicians.

- Wyatt's client base comprised mainly employers. Hospitals were clients, but only in their function as employers, so the focus was on employee benefits rather than on the care they delivered. Wyatt has tried to start a provider-based Health Care Consulting Practice without success. Other accounting firms, such as Ernst and Young, have had considerable success offering provider-based consulting to hospital and managed care accounting clients.

- Consulting work comes in cycles. If you are not busy with client work, sales and marketing fill your day. When these sales efforts yield more clients, billable client work mushrooms, precluding any further sales and marketing. So the typical practice veers between extremes of frantic client project work and sales and marketing to generate new projects.

For physician managers, consulting offers many good opportunities. The work is truly interesting; each project is substantially different than previous engagements. Clients need to be listened to carefully, their objectives and priorities clearly understood. The derived solutions will be idiosyncratic. There is an opportunity to work as part of a multidisciplinary team, which broadens the outlook on the entire project. The compensation level is very generous, probably greater than all but the most senior levels of management in managed care plans or hospital systems.

Consulting has its negative aspects, too. Travel requirements are huge. Two strategies that may reduce the required travel are to acquire a major client that anchors your consulting practice, reducing the amount of travel elsewhere, and to restrict your geographical range to a defined region (hard to do, especially in boutique or niche consulting).

There is a natural tension between consulting as a team, bringing more intellectual resources to a client at much greater cost (a higher hourly rate to bill the client), and consulting as an individual, which depends on one's own skills and experience (and being able to sell them), delivered at a lower cost (surprisingly, a lower hourly rate is much more profitable if the overhead is kept at a minimum). Each physician consultant must be comfortable with his or her position on this spectrum.

In employee benefit consulting firms, there are few colleagues and limited data and software resources. In these environments, a physician consultant must be comfortable with the lack of defined role models and be able to establish a path, using his or her own vision and the limits of available resources. In firms with large numbers of provider clients, health care consulting practices will have more physician consultant colleagues, more physicians in practice leadership roles, and greater access to sophisticated data sources and software. Again, one's comfort level with individual risk, the need to work in consulting teams, and the availability of role models will influence the type of consulting firm that seems the most attractive.

Value Health Sciences

In December 1993, I joined Value Health Sciences (VHS) as Medical Director. Based in Santa Monica, California, VHS makes clinical informatics and software tools that measure the appropriateness of diagnostic or therapeutic procedures, that profile physician practice patterns, and that serve as the clinical underpinnings of the Clinical Management System, the disease management system developed for the pharmaceutical giant Pfizer.

I was a virtual employee, in that I lived and worked out of a home office in Concord, Massachusetss, and traveled about half time to California to visit VHS, to New York City for meetings at Pfizer, and nationally for sales and marketing presentations with the Pfizer field force to prospective clients. My principal client was Pfizer. I helped it on strategy and tactics to roll out value-added services to managed care, physician group, employer, and business coalition marketplaces. My relations with Pfizer and its prospective clients were profoundly influenced by consulting experience gained at the Wyatt Company and in previous positions. My work with VHS taught me how to operate in a virtual environment, using a home office and modern technology to communicate with friends, prospects, and clients.

Independent Consulting

In August 1997, Value Health Sciences, as part of Value Health, Inc., was acquired by Columbia/HCA. Simultaneously, Rick Scott was replaced by Thomas Frist as CEO of Columbia, which decided to put Value Health up for sale. The ownership and business strategy of Value Health Sciences became unclear, and I was released by Value Health Sciences.

This opportunity allowed me to do what I had dreamed of doing: form my own independent consulting company, called Integrity Consulting, Inc. I have secured long-term contracts with a major pharmaceutical company and a start-up physician practice management firm, so my financial health is ensured for now. I am looking to add a third significant client and then will focus on delivering superb consulting and service for my three anchor clients. Later, if the opportunity presents, I would consider adding clients and the help of other consultants.

My experience as an independent consultant has validated what I have believed all along: smart and proactive organizations are very interested in gaining access to physician consultants who bring to the table clinical skills, business knowledge, expertise in information systems and quality measurements, and broad strategic and operations management experience. As the marketplace evolves and more physicians are willing to take the risk of becoming consultants, the opportunity for physicians to serve as skilled consultants will increase dramatically.

Conclusion

In summary, health care consulting for physician executives is a challenging and rewarding effort for conscious risk-takers. This practice exists on the boundary between domains of traditional physician influence in the health care delivery system and domains that significantly shape the delivery system—employers and their agents, payers, and managed care plans. The opportunity for a physician consultant with management training and experience to help rationally shape the health care delivery system cannot be overstated.

Chapter 7

Pharmaceutical Company Marketing Executive

by Geoffrey C. Porges, MBBS, MBA

As an aspiring physician, I was never really a good fit. When distinguished academic specialists approached me as a resident, offering the Faustian bargain of working on their service for a seemingly interminable number of years in return for a shot at the brass ring of their career, I somehow failed to get excited. But friends who had started their own businesses, or who had become journalists, or who ran for higher office—now there was a career! Nevertheless, I loved many aspects of clinical medicine and miss those aspects today—dealing with a wide variety of people one on one; really helping people in an hour of need or even crisis; and, finally, the intoxicating ego gratification of being one of the chosen brotherhood called doctor.

The Journey Begins

Over the past 10 years, I have moved from clinical medicine to pharmaceutical marketing almost by happenstance. That journey, and my responsibilities and activities in my present career, may be of some passing interest to the apparently growing number of dissatisfied medical graduates and physicians.

On some level, I was always uncomfortable with the detachment required for clinical judgment and with the deification accorded the medical profession. In some way, I recognized that information science could ultimately manage clinical decision-making far better than I. Personally, I was also too restless to want to stay in one hospital or one practice my whole career. In my formative 20s, I wanted to have a broader impact, to have more options, choices, and variety than I could find in clinical medicine.

Serendipitously, after three years of residency, the state health department where I lived precipitated serious thought on my part by advertising a medical management fellowship. In considering the fellowship, I recognized that the combination of business training and my medical education might allow me to meet more of my career interests. At the same time, I became enamored of my wife-to-be, who was about to begin her internship at a medical center in New York City. Through her academic colleagues there, I heard about a whole new industry, "biotechnology," based on exciting science and excitable investors. To the horror of family, friends, and interested bystanders, I followed that most important of all influences on any serious and successful career, being "in the right place at the right time," and plunged into the world of business.

When, in this way, I became a "management consultant," there were very few physicians in the field. Some had started but, failing to encounter the status, respect, and immediate lucre to which they were accustomed, had fled back to clinical medicine. These days, they might migrate the other way. At any rate, a rapidly growing, entrepreneurial, medical industry consulting firm called The Wilkerson Group took a chance on my business judgment and offered me an entry-level position in its technology and market analyst ranks. Shortly thereafter, I found myself on the phone day after day talking to academics, practitioners, investors, and even competitors about the next best way to cure metastatic renal carcinoma, disseminated lupus erythematosis, and other such serious conditions newly, and apparently miraculously, susceptible to technology-based therapeutic advances. What amazed me was that, after this cursory work on my part, senior managers in investment banks, venture capital firms, biotechnology companies, and ultimately even major pharmaceutical companies would listen to my assessments of their technologies and products and, in some cases, even act on those assessments! Once in a while, when I found technology that had a glimmer of reality and could be applied to a genuine and compelling clinical need, I could see impact of a breadth far beyond my original clinical background!

After several years as a consultant, serving clients as divergent as a global brewing company with money to burn in biotechnology and a syringe manufacturer looking at disease detection in saliva, I encountered a new obstacle. It was clear to me that the most important business decisions were usually made by the people who watched and counted the money, be they investors, division managers, or CEOs. And those people, for the most part, were not clinicians or scientists, but business people. I could win the trust and respect of the former, but the business people finally took their own counsel. I knew I could do what they did, but somehow, culturally, I had to "become one of them" as much as I was a physician. The shortest route to that was an MBA. And as much as there is an academic hierarchy in medicine, so there is a hierarchy in business schools. Each school has a brand as strongly as BMW and Chevrolet have distinctive identities. What better institution than the original MBA brand, Harvard Business School!

I suppose luck follows the brave, or the foolish, and after I persuaded my wife to leave New York for Boston and persuaded Harvard to have me, I found that Merck & Co., had an interest, at that time, in people like me. P. Roy Vagelos, MD, and I have very different educational and professional backgrounds, but somehow he believed that MD/MBAs would be valuable additions to Merck's management ranks. I hope he still thinks so. Merck and my wife both took chances on my skills and substantially supported my management education, then and now, for which I am very grateful.

As consulting taught me about the health care industry, Harvard taught me about the world of business. If anyone is torn between full-time and part-time school and can possibly afford full-time study, I would recommend it strongly . It is the difference between complete immersion and a series of short dips. At business school, I learned how the world of economics and industry operated, how to use the language of business, and which tools and techniques I could use in my career. I developed a network of colleagues who now populate the health care industry, and I developed relationships with distinguished and thoughtful teachers.

Where Can the Path Lead?

After business school, I saw, for almost the first time, the full range of opportunities open to me and also what opportunities I wanted to pursue. For me, the biggest thrill in business is making decisions about organizations, people, and products that improve, over time, the dreaded "bottom line." But the biggest thrill for me in medicine is making decisions that, over time, improve people's lives. In a leadership position in the medical products industry, at a sound and ethical company, I can do both of these things at the same time. I see science that often exceeds even the bounds of imagination in its potential impact and rewards. I work with leaders in clinical and academic medicine, and I contribute to a business that generates billions of dollars of value for shareholders, as well as for society.

As a leader in a worldwide marketing organization focused on vaccines, I now have a diverse set of responsibilities. First and foremost is functional expertise. I have to be effective in identifying market issues and opportunities and in developing responses to them. Internally, I also have to understand the processes and tasks of marketing management. What are the elements of a sound marketing plan, what constitutes good promotion, how can market research be structured effectively, and what key alliances and organizational changes are needed for us to achieve our business objectives? Marketing is about persuasion. At its core, my organization needs to communicate effectively the unique clinical; societal; and, increasingly, economic benefits of our products. The effectiveness of that communication is measured by changes in behavior that translate, ideally, into increased use of, or preference for, our products.

On a day-to-day basis, much of what I now do is managerial and administrative. One individual alone can accomplish very little in the marketplace, but if the 50 or 60 people in an organization are effective and their activities are more or less coordinated, we can really make things happen. Much of my work is now involved with the day-to-day business of managing the organization. Recruiting new talent to our organization; providing feedback to existing staff; and presenting new ideas, processes, and procedures to coordinate our activities occupy much of my day. In addition, I attend the usual series of management meetings. As the responsible marketing head, I need to represent my organization, and indirectly the customer, in discussions about product development, clinical trials, manufacturing plans, new dosages, product forms, and indications. Sandwiched between those major activities are tracking sales of our key products and striving to maintain both my background scientific knowledge and the customer contact that is critical to my role.

Looking at my current position and comparing it to clinical practice, I spend much more time in meetings and on airplanes. I often have to consider trade-offs that clinicians would consider unthinkable. (Should we pursue a malaria vaccine, for example, instead of improving an existing pediatric product?). My hours are generally more predictable than those of my friends in private practice, although frequent domestic and international travel probably makes up the difference. I rarely face the prospect of after-hours emergencies, but dealing with information and work overload keeps me occupied into the night anyway.

Inevitably, there are compromises in any career choice. Do I have to deal with bureaucracy and corporate politics even more than those that plague my wife's hospital practice? Undoubtedly. Are the financial rewards as attractive as those of many medical specialties? Hardly. But if, like me, someone is interested in the grand design of a business, the flow of industry, the massive and remarkable achievement of bringing new products to market, as well as emerging trends in biomedical science and clinical practice, medical technology companies are a wonderful place to be.

Opportunities, Lessons and Land Mines along the Way

In this journey of mine, what opportunities, lessons, and landmarks would I identify?

The most important question seems to be the one that I always ask physicians from anywhere when they ask me about jobs in industry. What do you want to do? What interests you, excites you, motivates you? If it's only a safe harbor, forget management. Business today is still at least as tough as clinical medicine and probably always will be. Money, too, is not enough. It is given even more sparingly to business executives than to physicians. If at all possible, physician executives should consider their ultimate goal before going to business school. That may influence the choice of school, the type of program, the projects and assignments selected, and the positions ultimately sought.

If someone really wants to get to a leadership position in a medical products company, whether it be diagnostics, devices, or drugs, he or she, regardless of medical training, needs to serve time in the management trenches. When trained physicians ask about joining our organization in an immediate leadership role, I ask them whether one of the newly minted MBAs in our marketing department could immediately assume leadership responsibility in their practices. Of course not, and the reverse is true. It takes time to learn how to analyze a market, build a forecast, write a marketing plan, develop a promotional campaign, manage a budget, or develop a team. All those years on the phone, analyzing markets and writing and rewriting reports and presentations as a consulting analyst, taught me valuable skills I still use today, skills that I did not learn at Harvard or in my residency. Somewhere, physician executives need to gain that initial experience in a company. Here are my guidelines for successfully making the transition to industry:

- **Choose Culture Carefully.** Choose a company that has physicians in senior business positions, not just research, otherwise you will be an obvious and temporary exception. Get to know those individuals and ask about their career paths and experiences. In fact, there are more physician executives than are readily apparent. Most of the more senior ones do not have MBAs, but they have extensive experience on the business rather than the research side of the company. Over time, they have learned not to advertise their professional training too widely. Follow their lesson!

- **Check Your Ego at the Door.** Being a physician is intoxicating, and the more clinical experience you have the more of an ego you may have developed and the more socialized to the role you are likely to be. Why do you think so many of your friends are physicians? To an extent, this pedestal is what people expect of their physicians, but it is not what people in companies expect from their colleagues. In my experience, the single biggest reason for failure among would-be physician executives is their lack of humility. Everyone, from the janitor to the CEO, not just your immediate peers, deserves your respect and recognition.

- **Expect and Accept a Step Down.** If you are serious about making a career transition into industry, you will have to accept starting at a lower level than you had expected. You can anticipate that, over time, your medical training will allow you to advance faster than your colleagues, but, initially, swallow your pride and learn the business in a low-risk, low-profile position.

- **Prove You Can Make and Handle Money.** There are core skills and assignments in any company, whether the position is sales representative, key account manager, product manager, or business unit manager. These positions tend to be in the "line" organization that actually carries the sales and income objectives for the business. In the long run, to be successful in any business environment and to achieve increasing responsibility, you have to prove yourself in one of these positions. In these positions, you learn how the company makes money and how to make decisions about what to spend money on given the many competing priorities. Find one of these positions and excel at it.

- **Find and Cultivate Mentors.** Mentors may be in the company or just in the industry, but when you meet a senior person with whom you connect and who is willing to support you, keep in touch. Whether contact is by occasional phone calls, lunches, cards, or whatever, these individuals will give you good advice and will help you advance in your organization and the industry.

- **Avoid Making Enemies.** The health care industry is remarkably small and people change jobs all the time. Subordinates or peers could come back as your manager, or could one day be recruiting you into another position. Make sure they respect your work and values even if you were not best buddies. One day, you may really need that headhunter you didn't bother to callback. Remember that what goes around comes around!

- **Use Your (Uncommon) Common Sense.** Ultimately, what business managers want is sound judgment. This means making the right call on tough decisions more often than not. If you are right 70 percent of the time, you'll be doing well. The exciting thing about business is that no two situations are the same, and no one has a guideline or protocol for how you should make those tough decisions. But if you are thoughtful, can apply your business and medical training and your career and life experience, and know when to ask and whom to ask, you stand a better chance of getting it right than most people do.

- **Ask for What You Want.** If you can get enough familiarity with a company or industry to clearly articulate what you would like to be doing in 3-5 years and beyond, and mean it, you have a better shot at getting it. Sooner or later, if you are consistent, someone will have an opening or an opportunity that fits what you want. And if you have shown you have the skills necessary in addition to your medical training, you will probably get that position. If, on the other hand, you're all over the place—"I'm not sure, maybe medical information, maybe licensing, maybe marketing"—no one will really extend themselves for you and you will not come to mind when any one of those positions becomes available. The person who really wants marketing will get that job and similarly for other areas.

- **Be Careful about Perceptions.** If you enter an organization in clinical research or academic affairs or business development, chances are that is how the organization will perceive you even if you had extensive marketing experience previously. If you want to work in a particular area, for example marketing, take a position in marketing, regardless of the level, rather than in a related area. That way you will demonstrate first hand your marketing skills and will be considered for more senior marketing positions later on.

Conclusion

These guidelines may seem self-evident or hackneyed, and to an extent they are. And most of them apply just as much to nonphysician managers and executives as to physicians. But it is amazing how many bright, ambitious, capable, aspiring physician executives ignore some or all of them and fail in a new position or organization. These are the rules everyone else learned from the school of hard knocks, and physicians often fail to pick them up in medical school. If you follow most of them, most of the time, you should ultimately achieve the success your extensive education, training, and investment deserve. Good luck!

Chapter 8

Outcomes and Health Policy Researcher

by David B. Nash, MD, MBA, FACPE (Hon.)

In researching and writing my first book in summer 1985, I coined a term that would help focus the next dozen years of my professional life and propel others to explore the MD-MBA pathway. If you read the overview chapter in the second edition of *Future Practice Alternatives in Medicine,* you will stumble upon the "white-coat/blue-collar" syndrome. In 1985, I began to wonder what the future of physicians' work would be like and was formulating my own career trajectory. In the pre-national managed care era, years before President Clinton's election, I was concerned about a class system for doctors—employee physicians and manager physicians. I had a sense that, as the marketplace matured, there would be distinct roles for physicians within management as well, a type of managerial specialization. I knew that I wanted to be a part of this burgeoning managerial class for physicians and was frankly very concerned about the assembly line-like work that I saw the early HMO models employing with physicians.

But, to put the white-coat/blue-collar syndrome into a context, I need to go back to my senior year in high school in spring 1973. With the reader's forbearance, let me trace my career trajectory over the past 20-plus years and in so doing elucidate the role of the policy maker and outcomes researcher who happens to be armed with an MBA degree. Simply put, an MBA alone is not the answer. The reader needs a context in which to place graduate management training for physicians.

High School Years

As the son of an entrepreneur and an elementary school teacher, I had no immediate physician role models in adolescence. Books and magazines in our home included *Forbes and Business Week,* and there were regular discussions about front-page stories in the *Wall Street Journal.* My high school was a very competitive one in an ethnically homogeneous area of southern Long Island, New York. Most of my contemporaries were interested in becoming physicians, propelled by their parents, a sense of future security, peer pressure, or some combination of those three. I had the intellectual engine to compete effectively in high school but never felt that I was a natural scientist capable of making important future discoveries. Of course, all career advice at that level was poor, if present at all. Remember, the television programs "Medical Center" and "Marcus Welby, MD," were helping to shape adolescent thinking about medicine in the early 1970s. Probably compelled by a mixture of an early interest in economics, an entrepreneurial father, and some sense that medicine would be an appropriate eventual career path, I began to think about what colleges to apply to on the basis of this odd mixture of emotion and analytic thinking.

In spring 1973, a few months prior to my graduation from high school, I read what would turn out to be the key article in my professional life in the metropolitan section of the daily *New York Times*. In this article, physician leaders of major New York hospitals were queried about their notion of what the future of medicine would look like. They described their own career paths and their trials and tribulations as major university-type hospital executive officers. I had, in retrospect, what one would call an epiphany reading this piece and recognized that this was the area I wanted to see myself in, in the very distant future—namely, physician director of other physicians. Certainly, I could not articulate that vision with any more precision in 1973. But I sensed that these men, and they were all men, had a grasp of medicine that I could not get from my own pediatrician or from other physicians I had either known, read about, or met socially. Buried deep in the article was a long quotation from a physician at the University of Pennsylvania who was heading up a then-new program in medical or health economics. The late Dr. Samuel P. Martin III was named at that time as the first director of the Leonard Davis Institute of Health Economics on the campus of the University of Pennsylvania's Wharton School of Business. Sam spoke of a vision of physician managers trained for leadership positions in hospitals and other health care settings in the future. Naturally, the article made no mention of managed care medical directors, the National Committee on Quality Assurance, report cards for physicians, or any of the modern tools of medical management.

Intrigued by this article, and probably filled with adolescent arrogance, I wrote to all of the physicians quoted in this rather extensive piece, having gotten their addresses by calling their secretaries at each of the dozen or so named hospitals. All of the physicians in leadership positions wrote me interesting, but probably perfunctory letters, making broad suggestions about what I ought to pursue in college and even which college I might attend. One physician, amazingly enough, responded to my letter by telephoning me at my home on Long Island and suggesting that I come and visit him prior to matriculating to college. Of course, that physician was none other than Samuel P. Martin III. And so, in late spring or early summer 1973, I visited Philadelphia for the very first time on my own to spend what would be a crucial and, in retrospect, "life-altering" afternoon with Sam in his office on the campus of the University of Pennsylvania.

Meeting Sam Martin, MD

It will be difficult for the reader to appreciate how quickly I can conjure up the emotion of that afternoon almost 25 years ago. Sam was an imposing figure, even at that time, standing at about 6' 4" and with a thick Missouri accent. He was like no other man I had met before. He spoke slowly and deliberately and seemed genuinely comfortable talking to a high school senior with gumption enough to write to him and to show up at his front stoop. Sam carefully probed (and I would come to learn many years later as a result of his own lifetime of analysis) my interest in medicine and in what was called at that time medical economics. He seemed fascinated by my description of the interplay of my father's entrepreneurial drive, my ethnic predisposition to medicine, and the obvious tension that I felt swirling around these issues. While I didn't really go to see Sam for answers, he provided many important answers at that fateful meeting.

For example, the *New York Times* article mentioned earlier failed to lay out an appropriate career trajectory for persons interested in leadership roles in medicine. In fact, it made no mention of graduate programs in health administration, combined degree programs in medicine and management, or other programs available even in 1973. Sam filled in these lacunae in my understanding in a non-patronizing and peer-like fashion. I was completely smitten with Sam's approach to my dilemma, which, at the time, I considered the most important, earth-shattering question that any high school senior was contending with. Sam laid out a plan. My recollection is that it did not matter which college I potentially would go to; he was interested in what I would major in and what my critical thought processes would be like. He wanted me to attend a school where I would have ample economic training, recognizing that all of the science would come later. Even at that early stage, he described a program to me that would later shape my life, namely, the Robert Wood Johnson Clinical Scholars Program that he was just beginning to head up at the University of Pennsylvania. He never mentioned an actual MBA degree, but he did say that there were appropriate pathways for physicians to combine their interest in medicine with advanced training in management.

He described the history of the Leonard Davis Institute and his hopes for training a future generation of physician leaders who would come to grips with the cataclysmic changes in health care that he was forecasting even at that time. This was all heady stuff for a high school senior, but it did make sense in an intuitive way, and I knew once I left Sam's office that I had stumbled upon the "Rosetta Stone" for my career. I knew that Sam had many of the answers, but he would not simply release the answer. He would make you stumble upon it and make you feel as though you had discovered the right answer. He was fond of saying, "I'm only here to open the doors; how you cross the threshold is up to you." Two decades later, I say the same thing to applicants to Jefferson Medical College and to internship and residency candidates at Thomas Jefferson University Hospital!

Strictly speaking, Sam gave no advice about which particular college to attend. His interest was in my pursuing opportunities for critical thinking. Having been graduated from a very large public high school on Long Island, I had many opportunities to attend a host of good undergraduate colleges or universities. I was able to narrow the search to schools that would enable me to focus on my early and undefined interest in medical economics. Fortunately, coming from an upper middle class background, my parents were able to afford virtually any school that I would have the grades and scores to gain admission to.

College Years

My parents made an extensive tour of the northeastern United States, including many of Ivy League and Seven Sister schools. At that stage of my life, I wanted to attend a school where few of my high school classmates would be. I wanted a college that had small classes, having experienced what it was like to be lost in a large introductory course during a summer exposure to Cornell University while still in high school. As a result of this somewhat negative experience in large classrooms and the need to be within a half-day drive from home, I finally selected Vassar

College in Poughkeepsie, New York. To many readers, Vassar evokes a century of female education and visions of Meryl Streep and Jackie Onassis. For me, Vassar was an important break with tradition from other members of my high school graduating class, and it represented a new frontier. My class represented the second fully coeducational class that Vassar would admit, having gone through a wrenching self-evaluation and a Board of Trustee-level decision not to merge with Yale University in New Haven, Connecticut. I arrived at Vassar in September 1973 with a class of nearly 500 students, many of whom, it would turn out later, were much better students than I.

Vassar is a relatively small college, with a total enrollment of just under 2,000 students. Without any graduate schools or professions schools, the faculty are free to concentrate on research and on undergraduate teaching. While certainly not a national scientific powerhouse, Vassar prided itself on small classes, with classroom participation by students being an integral part of the educational experience. Without fraternities, sororities, football, and other distractions, most of the student body were serious students interested in the liberal arts. Its country-like setting and century and half tradition made it an ideal place to pursue an eclectic course of study.

With the help of some enlightened faculty in the Department of Economics, I began to sculpt my earliest thinking about combining a career in medicine and a career in health administration. Even in a department with fewer than a dozen faculty, there were junior faculty in economics who shared my budding interest in understanding how the health economy worked. Although they conducted little or no research in this arena themselves, they were able to steer me to the professional literature and to faculty at other schools with interests in health economics.

Indeed, I credit my undergraduate advisor, Dr. Lawrence Herbst, whose enthusiasm enabled me to pursue essentially a double major in economics and premedical studies. At a small college, this double major posed some scheduling exigencies, as there were few sections of each required course available. Through it all, Professor Herbst was a good guide, excellent teacher, and eventually a friend. While I eventually achieved Phi Beta Kappa status in spring 1977, it did not come easily. I found that to compete effectively with my very bright classmates required hours of library work and intensive study habits. My fellow majors in economics expressed an air of benign neglect with regard to my interest in health care, but certainly I was free to pursue this early interest. In fact, I wrote my required senior thesis on the managed care industry. At that time, those words were not used to describe health maintenance organizations and as a result, I believe the title of my senior thesis was, "HMOs-Pandemonium or Panacea." In our senior required seminar course, which served as a thesis critique group, I became enamored of the early works of Mark Pauly and others who were just then staking out new territory in health care and medical economics. In 1977, I had never visited or seen a health maintenance organization, but work on my thesis convinced me that this system of health care payment might have some future merit. I only wish I had invested appropriately in the stock market and followed my hunch from academia to Wall Street!

Upon reflection, there was very little cross-fertilization in 1977 among the different departments at Vassar. The chemistry professors knew that I was an economics major, and they were sensitive to my needs but curious about my motivation. The standard premedical majors in biology, chemistry, and physics looked at me askance and wondered where my "true" interests lay. Even at that early stage, peer pressure was a powerful phenomenon that negatively shaped some of my views. In some quarters, there was outright distrust and animosity toward a non-bio major applying to medical school. Luckily, hard work, good mentoring, and high medical college admission test scores enabled me to secure entrance to no fewer than 10 schools by April 1977, just two months shy of graduation. At this juncture, a return to Sam Martin was certainly called for.

Medical School Years

While, at the time, I was bitterly disappointed that I had not gained admission to the University of Pennsylvania School of Medicine in order to be geographically closer to Sam, I was grateful to have a choice among medical schools. Sam felt that the strongest school was the University of Rochester School of Medicine and Dentistry and the Strong Memorial Hospital in Rochester, New York. He knew many of the faculty, especially a Dr. Ernest Saward, one of the earliest medical directors at Kaiser Permanente in California who had become an emeritus professor of Community Medicine at Rochester. This turned out to be a fateful connection. Sam felt that going to the strongest possible medical school would give me the greatest options in the future with regard to a potential career in academic medicine, government service, or the like. These were foreign concepts to me at the time, but I trusted his advice and eventually decided to attend Rochester. Rochester was built on one of the earliest medical school models and was populated by senior faculty from Johns Hopkins, Harvard, Yale, and other Ivy League medical schools. Rochester had a very small class of just under 90 persons and was considered a highly competitive school from an admissions perspective. In September 1977, I began my medical studies.

Very quickly, I learned that Rochester was nothing like Vassar. Our entire class of 90 stayed together all day in a traditional lecture room format with speaker after speaker trudging through what seemed an endless list of slides, formulas, and related minutia. By the end of the first semester in December 1977, I was ready to leave medicine and return full time to health administration studies. My grades were suffering and the prospects as I envisioned them then were bleak. Fortunately, other mentors emerged who, it seems to me now, Sam knew would help me maintain my inner compass. The late Dr. Robert Berg, Chairman of the Department of Community Medicine, and the late Ernest Saward, the emeritus professor noted earlier, prevailed upon me to apply for a special Rochester fellowship that was to be conducted at the Kaiser Permanente Health Services Research Center in Portland, Oregon. As a result of Dr. Saward's lifetime of service to Kaiser Permanente, the giant managed care organization had a commitment to Rochester medical students to provide a summer experience of research and work in the oldest and most famous health services research center in managed care.

I applied to this unique summer experience and was accepted by the faculty in Portland, Oregon. Therefore, in the summer of 1978, I had probably the key watershed experience that helped to shape my career in health services research, outcomes management, and the like. The Kaiser Permanente Research Center in Portland is one of the oldest and most respected independent health services research centers in the country. The founding director is an imposing figure both by reputation and by girth by the name of Dr. Merwyn Greenlick, known the world over as Mitch.

Mitch had a vision nearly 30 years ago that the Kaiser Permanente system provided a fantastic opportunity for population-based research. Indeed, the latent evaluative capacity of all of those charts for so many people over a long period would enable researchers, even in the pre-computer era, to make important inferences about how we can use resources in the most parsimonious way for the best possible outcomes for the largest number of people. Mitch, it appeared to me, single-handedly created the Portland Research Center and recruited PhD-level and MD-level researchers from around the country to share his vision of applied research.

Early in June 1978, Mitch laid out for me and my two medical student colleagues (the summer's three fellows) what our assignment would be. The goal was to think of a unique research hypothesis and then utilize the vast database of the Portland Research Center to derive some interesting and ideally publishable answers. We were aided in our nascent research effort by Rochester faculty who accompanied us to Portland, including the late Dr. Robert Berg and Dr. Robert Barker, one of the tenured physician faculty within the department. Again, the same pattern seemed to be displaying itself in my life that key mentors would have a critical role in shaping my early thinking about the health care system.

It was during that summer in Portland, Oregon, that I began to see first-hand, under the tutelage of Mitch and his peers, how managed care organizations actually worked. Dr. Donald Freeborn, the Associate Director of the Center, patiently guided me through my first scholarly work. I chose to help evaluate a recently created database of personal attributes of primary care physicians and what attracted them to work in the health maintenance setting. In retrospect, this database, which had been assembled in 1976, was at least two decades ahead of its time as we currently seek answers to the same questions; namely, what motivates physicians to do a good job in a prepaid setting such as Kaiser? Eventually, that paper was published in the *Journal of Community Medicine*,[2] but the main accomplishment of that summer was to cement my early thinking that research in this area could make an important contribution to medicine and to public health. I found experts and mentors who were enthusiastic about this kind of inquiry before it was popular. I found like-minded physicians who were excited about work in this arena and were unapologetic about their station in the academic hierarchy. I returned to Rochester for the second year of medical school invigorated and knowing that, although I could not yet articulate the role I would hope to play, this field would grow and nurture my budding interests.

The second year of medical school lay before me upon my return to Rochester in fall 1978. This seemed to me to be a general replay of the first year, with more classroom work, memorization, and rote regurgitation for exams. I hungered for the previous summer of stimulating independent inquiry on topics that seemed to be vastly more important. It was frustrating to have to memorize arcane equations knowing I had tasted another world of population indicators and seen how the preeminent managed care system of its time operated. The second year was an academic struggle but fortunately was highlighted by meeting my future physician wife at a medical student conference at the Mount Sinai Medical School in New York City.

Without dwelling on personal details, suffice it to say that Dr. Esther Nash would help focus my thinking in this arena and often times serve as my external barometer and guide to more real-world issues. By September 1979, I was anxious to approach the third year of medical school, don the white coat, and begin the process of what I viewed as the key two years toward becoming a "real" physician. The third year was a welcome respite from the classroom and convinced me that I had made the right decision in returning to Rochester that fateful December two years previously. By the end of the third year, the important internship decision was looming on the horizon and again I felt compelled to visit Sam and get his insight about clinical training and its long-term relationship to my further-refined career goals.

Residency Years

I returned to see Sam late in the third year of medical school to review opportunities for clinical training. My scores and medical school grades were good but certainly I would still be viewed as a nontraditional applicant, in much the same way that Rochester had viewed me three years previously. Sam again insisted that the actual site for training was not as important as the opportunities for critical thinking, mentorship, and building relationships with faculty. By this juncture, my relationship with him had passed the six-year mark, and I had no reason to doubt his excellent judgment. Esther, my wife by that time, also wanted an opportunity to study close to her parents in Philadelphia, and this became an important component in our collective decision making. Sam thought it would be good to return to Philadelphia, close to the University of Pennsylvania, so that our relationship could continue and he could further sculpt my thinking and bolster my eventual application to his program, namely, the Robert Wood Johnson Clinical Scholars Program.

Thus, by fall 1980, my wife and I found ourselves back on the interview trail, akin to what I had done for Rochester and Vassar almost a decade earlier. We were fortunate to be able to focus our collective sites on Philadelphia, thereby narrowing the field of potential hospitals for clinical training. With Sam's advice in mind, we interviewed at most of the university training programs in the Philadelphia area that were preparing house officers for careers in internal medicine. We narrowed our sights on the Graduate Hospital, at that time strongly affiliated with the University of Pennsylvania, because of its forward-thinking Chief of Medicine at the time, the late Dr. Philip Kimball. Kimball seemed to sense intuitively my interests and, although he was a subspecialist chairman, he understood how important medical economics and health administration would be to the future. Also, he was willing to make an important compromise and accept Esther and me as a couple outside of the National Residency Matching Program. As a result, fortunately, we knew that by accepting Graduate's offer for two internship slots, we would have secured our clinical training sites very early in the senior year of medical school. This enabled us to take care of important mundane details like searching for an apartment and moving our wares to Philadelphia earlier than our colleagues. We packed up a rented U-Haul truck of our worldly belongings and drove to downtown Philadelphia to begin our clinical training together in July 1981, just two short weeks after medical school graduation.

Internship and residency training in internal medicine in the early 1980s was characterized by the advent of AIDS, many months of intensive care unit exposure, and an overemphasis on passing the American Board of Internal Medicine certification exam. While I contended with these issues, other more important aspects of training began to impress me, namely, so-called system failures. We were repeatedly readmitting the same patients with asthma, congestive heart failure, diabetes, and alcoholism. We had virtually no outpatient follow-up for these inpatient problems. We were accountable only at the most basic level and had no control over the process of care that these patients encountered in the Graduate Hospital system.

I only learned years later that I contended with these system failures (special cause variation) by hiding and hoarding appropriate antibiotics, lumbar puncture trays, and the like in closets that only I was aware of. Unfortunately, every other house officer did the same thing to contend with system failures, and, as a result, we had a nonsystem! This only hardened my resolve that becoming a Robert Wood Johnson Clinical Scholar at the University of Pennsylvania, under Sam's tutelage, might somehow unlock the power to understand these system failures. Luckily, I applied early to the Clinical Scholars program and knew by the end of internship in July 1982 where I would be in July 1984, namely, entering the Wharton School on the campus of the University of Pennsylvania. And so, while my colleagues celebrated the end of residency, I was studying for the Graduate Management Admission Test, hoping to secure my place in the Wharton School. Still, I had realized a 15-year old dream to become a Clinical Scholar at Penn under Sam's tutelage. Finally, my formal MBA education would begin.

Fellowship Years

Reentering the classroom setting was a double shock. I had been ill prepared to face homework, tests, and classroom note-taking after three years of grueling residency training. I was in with a very elite group of peers in the Clinical Scholars program and the Wharton Health Care majors group. The curriculum, however, was very stimulating and, finally, it seemed to me, we were studying issues that had originally peaked my interest back in Portland, Oregon, during the experience at the Kaiser Permanente Research Center. Here were tenured professors studying health economics, professional liability reform, health maintenance organizations, and the like. The classroom work was challenging, and the group exercises required of all Wharton graduate students were daunting. During the summer between the two years of Wharton, I edited *Future Practice Alternatives in Medicine*, referred to earlier. The Wharton experience sharply focused my thinking about medical economics and the health care marketplace. Finally, we were learning the tools that I had hoped would enable me to make some future contribution to the health care system.

Contemporaneous with my last year at Wharton, I was selected as deputy editor of the prestigious *Annals of Internal Medicine*, published by the American College of Physicians in Philadelphia. Therefore, during my second and final year of MBA education, I shuttled back and forth between ACP headquarters, then in west Philadelphia, for two days a week and concentrated on my MBA studies the other three days. This hectic schedule broadened my horizons. I became one of the "best read" physicians in my peer group serving as secretary to the editorial board of the nation's third largest scholarly medical publication. The experience at ACP also taught me how little my senior colleagues knew about the functioning of the health care marketplace and how poorly prepared they would be for the cataclysmic changes shortly to come.

Did business school change my life? Indeed it did! It finally gave me the opportunity to spend sufficient intellectual time studying medical economics and appreciating the fund of knowledge and scope of the challenges before us. Wharton's emphasis on the free market and its expertise in finance, in particular, gave me a deep appreciation for the insurance industry and how payment mechanisms influenced doctor decision making. Through the faculty of General Medicine at the University of Pennsylvania Medical School, where the Clinical Scholars program was also based, we were exposed to some of the early giants in the field of applied health services research. Physicians such as Drs. John Eisenberg, Sankey Williams, and Sandy Schwartz were regular teachers, commentators, and research helpers to the Clinical Scholars. Sam's overriding, but unobtrusive, influence was everywhere as we sought answers to questions he had asked decades earlier.

Post-Fellowship Years

Upon graduation from the Wharton program in 1986, I continued on as a junior faculty member at the University of Pennsylvania School of Medicine. I kept my *Annals* appointment, at various times worked in the General Medicine unit at the Philadelphia Veterans Administration Hospital, and took charge of a nine-physician faculty group practice known as the Health Evaluation Center. These early managerial experiences were a testing ground for my new-found MBA knowledge. I quickly learned, as most MBA graduates do, that classroom learning has little application to managing physicians. I understood, at a front-line level, how difficult it was to motivate my colleagues to be more self-evaluative about their work and to be more accountable to their peers and to the payers of medical care.

Even in 1987, a decade ago, I saw how difficult it was to improve our day-to-day functioning without the tools I had learned at Wharton. Getting other physicians to think in a systems format was nearly impossible, as the cultural rift between us was so great. Remember, medical school teaches us—one patient, one problem, one at a time with the doctor at the center of the known universe. Modern management theory, of course, stresses the role of the system, with the doctor as a part, albeit an essential part, of that system. These early cultural conflicts continued to shape my thinking about what other contributions I could make to the health care system. I grew restless after nearly six years on the University of Pennsylvania campus.

That restlessness would lead me to the final part of this chapter and to the most recent aspect of my work, namely, becoming the founding director of Thomas Jefferson University's Office of Health Policy and Clinical Outcomes. Again, key mentors seemed to point me in the right direction. By late 1989, I felt, for various political reasons and from a sense of wanting to manage my own unit, that it was time to leave the university. I sought advice from Dean Joseph S. Gonnella, one of the longest serving medical school deans in the country. He asked if I would come to Jefferson and begin to create a new academic unit that he and others creatively called the Office of Health Policy and Clinical Outcomes.

Dean Gonnella knew that Jefferson needed trained MD/MBA faculty interested in doing research and teaching in areas that were under-represented in the faculty at large. I wanted to make sure the unit had an operational home, and, thus, we were able to create a linkage to Thomas Jefferson University Hospital under the leadership of Thomas J. Lewis, the hospital's Chief Executive Officer. Over the past eight years, the Office of Health Policy has grown to an 18-person, full-time, independent academic unit reporting directly to the Dean of the medical school and to the Chief

Executive Officer of the university hospital. With the formation of the Jefferson Health System, a multi-institutional health care system covering metropolitan Philadelphia and its suburbs, it is my hope that the office will take on more of an analytic role for the center at large. With more than $2 million in outside support and a staff of senior physicians, pharmacists, analysts, and others, the office has become Jefferson's epicenter for work on practice guidelines, quality improvement, health policy, and pharmacoeconomics.

The Office of Health Policy and Clinical Outcomes is one of nearly two dozen such offices around the country. With its multidisciplinary staff, the Office has three main goals.

Goal number one is to educate medical students, trainees, and attendings, at all levels of the spectrum, on issues of quality measurement and improvement. In addition, we provide unique curricular resources for teaching the tenets of managed care.

Goal number two is to do research in managed care, pharmacoeconomics, practice guidelines, and related areas. Our health services research agenda is broad and our articles have appeared in many different peer-reviewed and nonscholarly journals. We have prepared reports for organizations as diverse as the American Association of Retired Persons (AARP) and the National Association of Manufacturers in Washington, D.C.

Our third goal is to provide operational advice to both the hospital and the medical school in the areas of quality improvement. This means that I serve on numerous committees, at both the medical school and the hospital level, on quality. Again, as the Jefferson Health System matures, I believe the Office is perfectly suited to continue its analytic role and its research role. I am confident about our future growth and ability to contribute to the system at large. I hope that our system CEO, Doug Peters, shares this vision!

Not a day goes by, in my current role as Associate Dean for Health Policy and Director of the office, in which I fail to think of the lessons learned at Wharton and the cultural rift between medicine and management. The lessons learned from Sam Martin almost 20 years ago echo in my ears daily. In my view, only as physicians assume more managerial responsibility will we have an opportunity to change the system for the better.

I am grateful to be able to say that I probably would not have changed anything in a substantive way looking back on my career trajectory thus far. I am grateful to early, middle, and late mentors who guided my decision making from high school to college, medical school, residency, and beyond. I admire the leadership of the Jefferson Health System as it tries to forge new models based on cooperative arrangements with physicians, collegiality, and trust. Through it all, each day I look at the portrait of Sam Martin hanging on my office wall, and I think back to probably his most famous saying, which is etched in my memory forever: "How do you make a silk purse out of a sow's ear?" Answer: "Start with silk sows."

References

1. Nash, D., Editor. *Future Practice Alternatives in Medicine.* New York, N.Y.: Igaku-Shoin, 1993.

2. Nash, D., and others. "A Study of Physicians' Receptivity to Special Programs for Sociomedical and Behavioral Problems." *Journal of Community Health* 7(4):239-49, Summer 1982.

Acknowledgement

In addition to the individuals mentioned in the text, I want to thank my parents, Al and Charlotte, for all of their support and encouragement. Of course, my wife Ester, twins Rachel and Lech, and our son Jacob make the the entire journey worthwhile.

Chapter 9

Managed Behavioral Health Care Organization Medical Director

by David Whitehouse, MD, MBA, ThD

The sun is still contemplating raising its head over the horizon when the alarm goes off. I am in the hotel I always stay at when I come to Minnesota from Connecticut in order to be at corporate headquarters. Somewhat reluctantly, but necessarily, I move from the bed, switch on CNN news, and plug in the computer. I am waiting for the weather report. This is Minneapolis. If the day unfolds as it should, I have a 2:30 flight to Burlington, Vermont, through Philadelphia. The appointment was set up over a month ago and will be a two-day brainstorming session among the regional care center director; clinical care managers from our regional office in Lutherville, Maryland; myself as the medical director of the company; and a representative of PKC, a software developer with a leading edge program in "expert" diagnostic and clinical management capabilities. The program will play a pivotal role in standardizing and improving the quality of our clinical care management process if the launch of the pilot program in Baltimore goes really well. This is to be the first of joint application development (JAD) sessions that will aim at teasing out the subtleties and structure of the thought processes, conscious and unconscious, that lie at the heart of clinical decisions about diagnosis, treatment, and patient education and that are central to excellence in care management and our interaction with our providers.

Whatever the rhetoric of our discussions, our mission is clear—to bring to the provider/patient relationship a valuable resource and capability that was not easily available in the traditional roles of the past. Our task in care management is to add value to patients and providers. For providers, the task is to make available perspectives they might not have considered or information about treatment options they might not have had time to review in the hectic pace of their schedules. It is to add awareness of the practical availability of treatment options, along with information about support groups, patient education materials, etc. in the community, on the web, locally and nationally. It is also about letting providers know and examine for themselves the reliability and the validity of the information or opinions that we are sharing so that they can make informed decisions in the best interests of their patients. For patients, our role is to address their needs, to help them connect to the best resource for them by clarifying the scope of need, and to present them with options—treatments, providers, or facilities—that are researched and supported by solid data. The task is to help informed patients make the best decisions for themselves and to make the naïve patient better informed and more empowered.

I am excited about what we are doing, and I am always searching for ways to have an impact on the care that patients receive. To me, no different from the days when I learned my skills as a medical student or resident or practiced the art and science of medicine directly, each patient encounter raises the question: "What would I want done for me, or for someone I loved?" When I was a provider, at the end of the day I wanted to go home and feel that I had done the best, really the best for my patients. I think about the supports that would have helped me, and I want to make them available to my colleagues.

Last weekend was Easter, and, in Connecticut, the days were balmy, with the promise of long-expected spring. But April is not coming in like a lamb. The northeast is blanketed with a blizzard. This morning I will be involved in the weekly executive meeting in Minneapolis and by 5 p.m. tonight I will be negotiating delays and cancellations in the Philadelphia airport on the way to Lake Champlain. Finally arriving in yet another home away from home, I will check my e-mail from afar and close the office for the day after completing the executive summary for the antidepressant study in Massachusetts.

Medical School and Residency

Traveling to Vermont is always a bit like coming home. It was here that I worked in the Northeast Kingdom as the sole psychiatrist for one quarter of the state as payback for my National Health Service Corps scholarship, and, as I drive through the University of Vermont, I think back to my medical student days at Dartmouth and realize my career has unfolded in a way that I had never thought possible. I had come to medical school convinced that I would become a family practitioner. I had wanted to be the total doctor, taking care of all the needs of patients and their families. In a way, medicine was a natural progression from the theological studies that had preceded it. It was still about ministry but more focused. But this was the last of the three-year programs and the pace was hectic. A desire for family practice was gradually replaced by a genuine love for the field of psychiatry and the way that it seemed to capture the total spectrum of biological, psychological, and social factors that impinged on the health of an individual. Psychiatry seemed to require a Sherlock Holmes-like ability to attend to detail (the last medical consult) and a comprehensive overview that saw the patient as a member of a family, as part of a community system (a perspective and a skill that are not without their uses as one moves into the arena of health policy).

But time for reflection was limited. While some of my favorite memories of those days may have been afternoon tea in the classic surroundings of the Sanborn library, creating a respite from cramming for a dermatology or hematology final, clinical rotations jumped rapidly into the picture. And the nature of the three-year program was that residency choices had to be made with only two clinical rotations under our belts. So it was with my knowledge of the world of medicine still remarkably limited in scope that I found myself bound for Boston and Massachusetts General Hospital (MGH). Earlier in my life, I had considered ordination and came to the United States from England at 24 years of age to read theology at Harvard.

"Medicine, religion; religion, medicine. It seems that you have had a hard time deciding which has the greatest magic," the admissions interviewer had asked. "And the jury is still out," I had replied. The world of corporate medicine was the farthest thought from my mind. In fact, I remember that I had had a certain disdain in those Dartmouth days for colleagues who sat at the back of the lecture hall, seemingly more interested in the Wall Street Journal than in the mysteries of arthritis. I wanted to be the best clinician I could. I had chosen MGH in part because of its insistence on a solid medical internship and of its strong consultation service.

Now it was residency and, if internship had been its own baptism by fire, the Acute Psychiatric Service at MGH was to be the ultimate testing ground. Logan Airport seemed to be a regular port of call for bipolar patients exercising their wanderlust, and the hospital itself was sufficiently accessible to make the emergency department a regular stop for a variety of recreational drug abusers, distressed individuals, and the tragic victims of abuse and rape. There was a consultation-liaison service; burn patients, oncology patients, the agitated, the detoxing, the abandoned, and the depressed. There was a chance to look at the total impact of illness in terms of behavioral medicine and medical psychiatry and at the impact of personality on patient and physician alike. But, for the most part, the focus was on treatment, triage, and sickness. The world of health promotion and prevention was a long way off. In the community-focused part of training in a clinic in East Boston working with the courts, the schools, and primary care doctors, there was a context for this world, but most of life was lived in the immediate, the acute. At the same time, however, more by accident than design, I was to get my first introduction to the world of health policy and management.

At the end of my first year at MGH, my residency training director nominated me for a position on the Committee of Residents for the American Psychiatric Association (APA). His kind words of recommendation must have carried the day. One night, while I was on call at the state hospital, the phone rang and I was informed that I had been duly elected to the Committee and was to start within a few weeks as resident representative to the Board of Trustees. As someone who had had a profound distrust of organized medicine, this was to be an awakening.

I will never forget the first meeting. With only days left before the meeting, major tomes of materials arrived, including minutes from various committees, action items from the Assembly, reports, and a draft edition of an entire work on the homeless mentally ill. Overwhelmed, I dutifully read it all, not knowing whom I might meet or why my opinion would be worth anything. I set off for Washington totally ignorant of what might be entailed. Accommodations were elegant (very) and in stark contrast to the on-call rooms I was used to, and my anxiety only heightened. The next day, I met the Board and realized several things: one, I was probably one of very few people in the room who had read every piece of material sent out; two, these learned colleagues, with their wealth of practical experience and academic wisdom, were interested in the opinions of those who would inherit the profession; and three, to be able to step back from immediate crises of individual cases and look at the broad panorama of one's profession—its scope, its mission, its challenges—this was exciting.

The second day concluded with the APA's legal team's discussing a brief in Florida that focused on an issue that would never have even crossed my mind, "competency to be executed." It was and is a bizarre Alice through the Looking Glass type of question. To participate in the debate was not only intellectually, professionally, and ethically demanding, but also helped me to understand for a moment that health care decisions could have widespread ramifications. The seeds of a future drive to make a difference at the macro level were sown.

Back at MGH, Chester Pierce would continue to challenge my thinking, whether discussing psychiatry and medicine from an anthropological perspective, discussing the challenges of manned space flight, or examining the American Bar Association's views on the death penalty. I found myself investigating and advocating changes in training, bringing together colleagues from around New England, discussing the process of what we were doing in training as much as the content. With this, my world view grew and I loved it. Within a year the medical student who would have nothing to do with the American Medical Association (AMA) was replaced by a resident running for the Governing Body of the AMA's Resident Physician Section. I was elected. Now, every month, I was at some meeting across the country, learning, challenging, advocating, defending positions on issues—issues of training, issues of discrimination, issues of services for our patients, and issues on health policy.

I was asked to serve on the AMA's Task Force on Physician Manpower. Here too, I was to experience a perspective I will not forget. The mandate was to create a comprehensive position paper on physician manpower issues within 12 months. There was a huge amount of information to be assimilated and debated. Nevertheless, we would meet just four times. The task seemed daunting. What I had failed to take into account were the skills, expertise, and energy of the staff people who crafted the drafts; did the research; and, more impressively, made all of their work accessible. One week before a meeting in Chicago, I had been reading a draft of one of the position papers and felt that there were perspectives on the role of physician extenders etc. that needed to be addressed. I called AMA and asked for some help researching the issues so I could add some value to the discussions later in the week. When I arrived at the hotel, there was a four-inch-thick pile of papers awaiting my perusal. The task seemed impossible until I read the covering note and saw that each paper had been annotated. "The graphs in this paper are excellent summaries but the topic is better discussed in the…article." The following day, I added value to the debate because that level of preparation created the perfect synergy. I don't have that available to me now, but I think of it often and wonder how much better some of our executive meetings might be if we came to them as prepared.

Early Experiences in Management

While health policy had now captured my imagination, my immediate career choices were not my own. In return for support during medical school, I owed the NHSC two years. So, while my colleagues were busy deciding how to leverage the excellence of the training program and their own unique gifts as they freely embarked on their professional careers, my journey led to Vermont and the Northeast Kingdom. In fact, this was to prove a perfect fit. As the sole psychiatrist for one quarter of the state, my role was not just clinician but "medical director." It was my first experience with the physician as manager. The issues the clinic faced were not just individual clinical problems but the delivery of mental health care in a rural area with limited resources. Protocols, quality improvement initiatives, training, supervision, regulatory compliance, vertical integration, horizontal integration, and primary care integration were all areas that fell under my responsibility. Like many physicians, my first training in medical management, therefore, came out of the practical realities of everyday life. My teachers were seasoned colleagues who had established and developed the system of care over years.

What is interesting to see now is that the model that we used more than 10 years ago out of necessity—a primary care delivery model in which simpler cases stayed with the family practitioners and more complicated ones belonged to the mental health clinic and in which the emphasis was on early intervention and alternatives to hospitalization—is now touted as the new integrated model of the future. At the end of the day, the rewards were twofold: individual cases for which good clinical care made a difference to specific patients and establishment of a way of operating a whole system of care that allowed the community to maximize the impact of limited resources. The problem for me was that the lack of support meant that I was on call 24 hours a day, seven days a week.

At the end of two years, my family and I moved back to Connecticut so that our children could be closer to their grandparents. Professionally, I had enjoyed the system challenges in Vermont, and so, as we moved south, I was looking for an opportunity to further develop the clinical medical management skills I had begun to use. In the city where we wanted to locate, there was an opening for a director of outpatient services at a large general hospital with a comprehensive private practice model department of psychiatry. The job was interesting enough in and of itself, but what made it more exciting was the possibility of putting in a brand new program, expanding the scope of ambulatory services, and creating a better delivery system. However, before I arrived to take the job, the chairman of the department resigned and in short order I found myself as chairman.

I had wanted a challenge but this was more than I had expected. JCAHO, state licensing, departmental committees, and budgetary processes all became part of the new repertoire. One of the more demanding tasks, however, was the whole question of how to work best in a private practice model. The greatest revenue generators for the hospital were often psychiatrists who had perfected the art of referral at the cost of the art of treatment. Referrals were frequently based on whom the referrer liked best, either because they were convenient (they never said "no"), as a quid pro quo (well you refer to me so I'll refer to you), or because the receiving doctor nurtured the relationship with the residents in the emergency department through whom most of the referrals came. If quality was poor but utilization patterns were high, the hospital might be more interested in your turning a blind eye. The tension between immediate economic success and the promotion of best practices was a dilemma that all department heads had to face.

Working to change and improve the practices of colleagues in order to raise the community standard was a new skill. Understanding how the department budget, the financial viability of the hospital, the needs of the patient, and the needs of the community acted as drivers on behaviors and decisions deepened one's understanding of the development of health policy. It soon became clear that we needed to develop a whole strategic plan to bring department, hospital, and individual goals in line, given the onset of managed care and the shifting realities of reimbursement. The strategic planning process was another first. The discipline of planning activity, its focus on data, highlighting of problems in data sufficiency, and integrity, led to new insights. Now, for the first time, I realized I needed more formalized training. Also for the first time, I became exposed to the American College of Physician Executives (ACPE) and its Physician in Management seminars (PIMS).

I had been excited about physician management before, but these seminars added fuel to that fire. The lecturers were, without question, the most dynamic I had or have encountered. Awareness gained in the seminars of how the skills that made one an excellent clinician—self-reliance, personal accountability, willingness to shoulder the burden alone, capability of making life and death decisions on limited data, and clinical wisdom—were often in conflict with the core skills of good management—the ability to empower a team, to delegate effectively, and to balance the trade-offs of short- and long-term goals—explained why the best clinicians do not necessarily make the best physician managers (although it is often the norm that physician management positions are given out as the reward for excellence in clinical skills).

At the same time, it was a great boost to meet and exchange ideas with other physicians who were taking the shift in roles and the need for new skills seriously. With this came the understanding that, for many colleagues and even family and friends, there was something suspect about the role of the physician executive. For many, the role shift was about turning medicine into a business. It was about killing the artistry, the wisdom, the caring of a noble profession and reducing it to the realm of case studies and business ethics. It was also about the struggle to integrate the personal caring of the physician and the qualities that had brought the respect of peers and family with this shift in roles and about overcoming the sense of suspicion and disappointment that the shift engendered in peers and family members. The Clinton health debate was just warming, and, although for me it highlighted the challenge of creating an accountable, affordable, and accessible health system, for many it seemed to highlight the split between the world of managed care, the business of medicine, and the calling of patient advocacy. Where I saw a common agenda, others saw dichotomy. At the PIM seminars, however, there was a common language, an excitement, and a respect for these new skills and the possibilities of what one could do in these new roles.

Back at the ranch, pressures on the hospital from local competition, reorganization, and downsizing meant that the overall impact of my strategic planning was minor. Now was not the moment, nor did it look like it would be for a while. As a result, when an opportunity presented itself across the border in Massachusetts, I went to investigate and saw in the challenge of this new situation a chance to hone the skills I had and develop new ones in solving problems and creating new health care solutions. Little did I know.

On the home front, we had made a decision. The children were happy with their school and the community. These new roles, unlike that of the independent clinician who establishes a community base and then grows old in it, seemed to offer less "permanence." What I translated as an "exciting challenge" was reframed as "potentially risky." If permanence seemed to advocate for relocation, risk seemed to suggest the need to maintain home life stability. The decision was made. I would commute, and they would stay put. With four children in private schools, (13, 10, 7, and 4), there is always somebody for whom the move would be bad. At the same time, especially as one moves up the ladder, jobs becomes scarcer.

Balance has been and is a major factor in maintaining and developing my career within the needs, dreams, and hopes of a family life in which children look to you for role models, support, and participation. At the same time, in a two-career family, the impact of any decision carries with it deep consequences for one's partner.

The flexibility to work from home, the era of the mobile office, and the power of electronic connectivity have all played a role in making the impossible possible. Nevertheless, to underestimate the impact of such a move on one's family and the significance of joint decision making and prioritizing would downplay the most vital source of energy and sense of self-worth that exists—one's role as spouse and parent.

Hospital Medical Director and CEO

I began the commute to the new job and entered a different state in more ways than one. The new job entailed being medical director of a start-up hospital that was to form the basis of a whole behavioral health care delivery system that would link with community agencies, home outreach, elder care, and school systems. It would respond to the cultural and ethnic diversity of the community. It would link to the core agencies of other hospitals, police departments, and social service agencies. It would take a brand new facility and create an environment in which public and private patients would feel at home. It would respect patients as individuals and service their physical and spiritual health as well as their psychiatric health. It would allow the state to close and then privatize the acute admitting and forensic units of the state hospital and to provide those services better and more cost effectively in a private setting.

This was health policy and strategy in the making. If the clinical challenge was enormous, the operationalizing of it was to be an eye opener. Clinically, one had to develop entire departments from scratch. Policies and procedures had to be developed to meet state, federal, and JCAHO mandates. Quality improvement training needed to be initiated and quality management and risk management programs put in place. All this had to be done while hiring key clinicians who would drive the success of the institution. Staffing had to be established that would allow for a gradual build up of census for full programming and safety while not taxing resources unduly. These were exciting days and the sense of creativity, challenge, and commitment ran high. Problems were encountered and overcome. Things appeared to be moving slower than we had hoped, but the future looked good.

After about 14 months, the CEO left to take a university post and with his departure came the opportunity to move from medical director to CEO and medical director. Never one to miss an opportunity to grow, I offered my services and was accepted. In retrospect, it was to be the beginning of the fastest professional growth curve I have ever had. It also helped better define for me what about medical management I really enjoyed and what about nonmedical management I had no passion for.

In the next few weeks, I was to discover that there had been issues with payroll taxes. As CEO, I was personally at risk for the taxes. I was also to learn that, as part of cash flow problems in a start-up situation, certain bills were prioritized over others and that there were vendors who needed to be dealt with. It was clear that our financial department was not doing the job we needed it to do, that our cost accounting capabilities were negligible, and that our information substructure was inadequate. At the same time, our involvement in closing the state hospital brought unprecedented oversight by state regulators and the media and considerable political posturing by friend and foe alike. These were new arenas of operation for me. Meanwhile the NIMBY (not in my backyard syndrome) was alive and well and causing its own share of pubic relations problems in the community. My business education began in earnest. First, it was education to survive and then education to succeed, and then, two years later, we had a superb onsite senior management team. We had taken a significant tax liability and completely resolved it. The institution had moved from the red to the black, and, along the way, I had earned an MBA.

When I was thinking about a career as a physician executive, I remember discussions with colleagues in the ACPE about the value or lack of value in getting another degree. Whenever I asked which degree would be best (MPH, MBA, MHA, etc.), the answer always was "it depends on what you want to do eventually." I can only speak to the MBA, but I am really glad that I chose it. I use the skills and the perspectives that I gained during the program daily. As I looked at MBA programs, certain things were givens: (1) it had to be accredited, especially if it was to be portable, and (2) it had to fit in my work schedule. Executive MBA programs tend to run on two schedules. Those that meet every other Friday and Saturday and those that have long residential periods interspersed with a lot of interactive work by phone and computer.

Regardless of which approach is selected, a significant commitment is required. The payback, however, is tremendous. One of the factors that was important to me was to be part of a program that involved more than health professionals. In executive MBA programs, as much informal learning takes place among group members as occurs in formal didactic sessions. In the two years that we were together, we went from being a group to being a team. We learned to trust each other, help each other, and enable each other. In my group was a senior executive from GE Capital, an engineer from Sikorsky, an advertising executive from Duracell, a senior payroll manager from IBM, and a young woman whose international experience included setting up three businesses in Moscow and the planning of a significant retail development connected with GUM, the famous Russian department store. We had finance, strategic planning, design, marketing, and sales covered.

The program was to be an insight into the corporate world that has served me well today, learning first-hand what was important and getting an inside look at corporate cultures very different from the world of medicine. At the same time, an unexpected awakening happened, in that the experience fired in me a real interest in international development that has become part of what I do today. In addition to rapid enhancement of computer skills that was necessary to survive, another bonus of this program was an international experiential module that occurred in the summer between the two years. During these 10 days, we went to Singapore and Hong Kong to learn first hand about the growing Asian economies. Finance and accounting were more challenging courses but, in the end, were the most rewarding. Further, understanding of group dynamics and leadership and management skills helped juxtapose the unconscious attitudes of the independent, autocratic, knowledge-rich physician against some of the team building, wisdom sharing, empowerment practices that are vital in successful businesses today.

Let's also be honest. It was also fun. Acting out the market problems of Dry Creek Vineyards, studying the decisions of Phil Knight as he brings Nike into the 21st Century, comparing annual reports and financial statements of Komatsu and Caterpillar, arguing the points of business ethics, and listening to the entrepreneurial plans of one's colleagues stretched the mind and, despite the hours, provided excitement and challenge. In addition to weekends, we would meet generally once a week at one another's work sites. The pressures of the regular work week and the need to maintain some semblance of family life required extraordinary flexibility at home and a genuinely supportive environment at work. At times, excitement in class would be mitigated by a crisis on the home front. At others, the exhaustion of an all-night session struggling with the problems of cost accounting would be compensated by the perspective of a birthday or school event. Training in the middle of one's career can be remarkably rewarding. The combination of maturity, experience, interest, and determination and perseverance of one's colleagues are an invigorating mix, but the commitment is not to be taken lightly.

Armed with these new perspectives and insights, I returned to my job with vision and purpose that drew energy from the challenges and saw new opportunities in my work. The strategic task at hand was moving beyond the early successes of the financial turnaround and building a future in a highly competitive health care environment. Knowledge about information systems and cost accounting became the focus of the reengineering effort. Work on integration, partnerships, and acquisitions filled the day. The clinical focus moved to the development of niche programs, cultural relativity, and standardization of process. Outcomes research, care mapping, CQI teams, and patient satisfaction were the cornerstones of the changed focus.

At the same time, the differences between the roles and responsibilities of the CEO and the Medical Director began to come into focus. For me, personally, this reached its culmination the day I spent with the police and the kitchen staff investigating the theft of chefs' knives from the kitchen. I realized that this was not the level of activity that inspired me. At the same time, the company was looking to reorganize, and, with our mutual destinies now getting ready to take different paths, I began to look for opportunities that best fitted my training, experience, and drive for opportunity and creativity. The tasks of solid financial management, successful privatization, program development, integration planning, and clinical improvement strategies gave me a solid foundation. As jobs appeared, it became clear that, whether it was in the arena of managed care, the pharmaceutical industry, or integrated delivery systems, the issues were the same—disease management, patient satisfaction, outcomes analysis, and episode of care or some other cost accounting analysis to support disease management. Managerially, I felt ready for a broader challenge, and, when the opportunity arose to join MCC Behavioral Care as national medical director, it seemed a perfect fit. Managing clinical delivery systems and care management systems on a national basis would require a new set of skills. Underwriting and risk-assessment skills would also be new. But the core skills necessary for the task—clinical wisdom and health strategy development experience—would be building on the competencies that I already had.

MCC (a subsidiary of CIGNA) has been one of the most exciting and compelling opportunities I have encountered. Clinical strategy development has brought me in contact with cutting edge developers of clinical information systems, intelligent decision support tools, outcomes instruments, and neural networks. The desire to collaborate with providers—be they hospitals, integrated delivery systems, groups, or individuals—has taken me into the field, listening to providers' issues, trying to better understand their work flows, and sharing with them excitement for the opportunity to get fast reliable feedback and benchmarking capabilities. Quality imperatives have led to involvement with accreditation agencies and to reengineering of our clinical outcomes' study process and design. Health policy and strategy improvement has led to work on multisite studies with academic partners and enlightened employers.

An unforeseen bonus has been the fact that CIGNA, by virtue of its global status, has afforded me the chance to work with international health opportunities as they have come up. Travel has become a way of life. Generally, I travel to three different ports of call per week. The travel is tiring, but the people, the encounters, the wisdom that come from the chance to really talk and interact with those who deliver care and care management on the front line, to hear customers' needs first hand, to understand geographic variation, and to see the real impact of the decisions we make are part of the life blood of management for me.

Conclusion

In some respects, my career has been a response to opportunity. In others, each stage has built on the skills and expertise of the previous chapters in my life. I know for certain that clinical thinking and health policy awareness that are fundamental in all that I do would not be there without the solid training and clinical wisdom I learned at Dartmouth and MGH. On top of this, my understanding of different delivery systems and the world of the provider has been enhanced by direct experiences I have had in rural care in Vermont, in general hospital private practice in Connecticut, in the private for-profit world of the integrated delivery system of Charles River Hospital-WEST, and in academic training centers at Dartmouth, Yale, and Harvard. The world of business and health policy development grew from those first experiences in organized medicine into the formal training of the MBA and has been seasoned by practical experience and corporate challenge. Caring about the health and wellness of individuals is the passion that drives it all. Yet all this takes place within a context, the context of a family which gives rootedness and stability to all the drive, passion, and challenge.

So my fellow management travelers, *carpe diem*, seize the day. After all, it is your future and the moment is now. Opportunities can slip away. For me, the excitement and the genuine joy of working in administrative medicine await. If you find yourself going my way, be in touch. Networking and mentors are key for growth in career development everywhere but especially in clinical administration.

Chapter 10

Information Systems Specialist

Marshall de Graffenried Ruffin Jr., MD, MPH, MBA, FACPE

My father practiced medicine. He finished Harvard Medical School in 1936 and pursued eclectic residency training that included one year of general surgery at New York Hospital; one year of emergency medicine at Emergency Hospital, Washington, D.C.; two years of pathology at Massachusetts General Hospital; and, recognizing he was most interested in mental health, a residency in neurology and psychiatry at the Hospital of the University of Pennsylvania. He practiced psychiatry and psychosomatic medicine in a group practice in Washington, D.C., before World War II, and, after the United States entered the War, he enlisted in the Army Air Corps and served as a flight surgeon in Texas and Florida. After the War, he returned to Washington, D.C., and completed analytic training to practice as a psychoanalyst. He practiced psychoanalysis and psychiatry for more than 30 years in solo practice in a row house near Dupont Circle that also housed the practices of two other psychiatrists and one general internist. For nearly 30 years, he taught an elective course in psychosomatic medicine at the George Washington University Medical Center. My father saw his last patient just a few months before his death from metastatic transitional cell carcinoma of the ureter on June 21, 1984. He was 72 years old when he died. He loved every moment of his work in medicine.

Emulating Dad

I wanted to be a physician, just like my father, when I was very young. I aimed my academic work at that goal. At the University of Virginia, I majored in chemistry and English. I did better in the sciences than in English, but I enjoyed English more than the sciences. At Harvard Medical School, I majored in the neurosciences, to be like Dad. While at Harvard, I took an elective in epidemiology and found it fascinating but of little interest to most medical students and faculty. I matched to Duke University Medical Center for a straight internal medicine residency. At Duke University, I enrolled in a program to earn eligibility to take the boards in medicine and neurology at the end of five years. But along the way, I found my interests in neurology waning and in economics and public health growing. I wondered how our country would pay for all the services I saw lavished on the dying and near dead in hospitals in Boston and Durham. I wondered why more incentives were not given to people to remain healthy. Prevention seemed to me to be far less expensive than treatment.

At the beginning of my third year of residency, I saw a poster for a Robert Wood Johnson Fellowship that would give me a fellow's salary to study public health and health services research for two years at one of several eminent medical centers, including the School of Public Health of the University of North Carolina, the University of Pennsylvania, Stanford University, UCLA, and the University of Washington. I was accepted to my first choice, the program at the School of Public Health of the University of North Carolina, Chapel Hill, just 10 miles from Duke. I made arrangements to complete neurology training at Duke after a two-year hiatus to learn about epidemiology, health policy, and economics at Chapel Hill.

My interest in computers started in high school, when, in 1969, the school offered a programming course in Fortran. As a senior, I used a precious semester elective to take the class and found it fascinating. We typed into a Teletype without a monitor and used paper tape to store our programs and our data. For my end-of-term project, I created a computer dating service for students in high schools in my community. I sold more than 500 questionnaires at five cents each and found underclassmen willing to enter the data into the Teletype. Several classmates more adept at programming than I helped me refine the program. When we ran the batch file with all the data entered, mysteriously I was matched to the two most beautiful girls in the senior class, with my favorite of the two listed first. And the system reciprocated by giving those two girls my name as their best match. Wondering at my stunning good fortune, I surveyed the data tape to find the programming logic that matched me uniquely to them, but never could detect gerrymandering of the program to my benefit. My friends denied any special programming on my behalf. They claimed that, had they modified the data to assign girls to boys, they would have matched me with my sister, not the girls the system assigned to me. The system helped me to arrange to date each girl to whom I had been matched. Needless to say, I was impressed with the power of computers to find valuable patterns in data and to do good for mankind.

Premed and Medical School

I graduated from high school in 1970 and attended the University of Virginia to earn my undergraduate degree in English. I minored in chemistry and took more than enough sciences to satisfy requirements of medical schools. I suppressed my continuing interest in computers to win a place in medical school. Many times, I considered taking programming courses but found other sciences and the humanities more interesting. In medical school, I took no time for computers but continued to read popular reports of improvements in their capabilities and of exciting prospects for their potential.

In my third year of medical school, during my internal medicine rotation at Massachusetts General Hospital, I was aware of computer monitors on the patient care units of the White Building, into which clerks entered orders we house officers wrote on paper, but I do not recall using those monitors. My interest in computers sparked when a gaunt fellow named Ted Shortliffe, MD, PhD, became my intern for one of those three months, and I learned that he had a doctorate in computer science. He described his work on MYCIN, an expert system to advise house officers in the selection of antibiotics to treat patients with meningitis. To my knowledge, we never used MYCIN at MGH, but suddenly I saw a whole new way in which computers could help doctors, by giving them advice. Ted was too busy being an intern to do much teaching about computers and medicine. I remember feeling strafed and humiliated by our attending, Gil Daniels, MD, a small, impatient endocrinologist, because of his disgust with me that I could not seem to remember the difference between systole and diastole. Even though Octo Barnett, MD, ran the Computer Science Laboratory at MGH and Ted Shortliffe, MD, PhD, was my intern, I did not seize the opportunity to rekindle my interest in computers. Instead, I retreated from my average performance on the wards and read Thomas Mann's *The Magic Mountain.* I was not a happy camper.

Residency at Duke

Oblivious to the significance of the advent of the personal computer, I finished medical school in 1978 and drove to Durham, North Carolina, to start my residency. At Duke, I learned about the Duke Cardiovascular Database, created at Duke under the direction of Eugene Stead, MD, who had built the department of Medicine at Duke and had only recently retired from the Chairman's position. His successor was James B. Wyngaarden, MD. The Duke Database kept detailed data from histories and physical examinations, cardiac catheterization studies, laboratory results, and surgical findings of myriad patients who moved through the medical center. As an internal medicine house officer, I observed the careful collection of data for the database and read the computer reports projecting patients' risks of subsequent cardiovascular ailments depending on whether they accepted medical or surgical therapy for coronary artery disease. As a medicine resident on cardiology I completed many of those survey forms. I read the interpretations of electrocardiograms performed by a large machine in the ECG laboratory and found them appropriate for most patients. Throughout my residency I retrieved detailed laboratory results on patients from text-based dumb terminals in work areas of patient care units, using a light pen to interact with the Duke Hospital Information System and the information system at the Durham VA hospital. I did not ask about vendors, or hardware, or networks. Those thoughts did not occur to me while I tried to learn internal medicine, but I noticed many signs that computers could facilitate the practice of medicine. I recall most the convenience and freedom given me when I could sit at a terminal and retrieve current and historical information on patients from monitors at helpful locations. I hoped I would have such devices in my office wherever I practiced medicine.

During my second year of residency, I met the second physician about my age who already had a doctorate in computer science. Alton Brantley, MD, PhD, was my intern on a medical service for which I was the junior assistant resident (JAR). JARs know everything, and interns know nothing. After sizing up Dr. Brantley and deciding that, because I was a JAR from Harvard Medical School and he was an intern from Duke Medical School, I was going to win any intellectual disagreements we might have, imagine my surprise to discover that he already had a doctorate in computer science. Not only did he understand the mechanics of the information systems that gave house officers data about their patients, he had participated in the design, development, and deployment of those systems. Duly humbled, I became a better house officer and thoroughly enjoyed my brief term with ever-cheerful and always inquisitive Alton. To my delight, in 1996, Alton and I began to work together at The Informatics Institute, of which he is a successful member of the faculty and of the Advisory Board. He works full time as Chief Information Officer of Medlantic Healthcare Group, based in Washington, D.C.

Early in my JAR year, my father called me to let me know that he had noticed hematuria and that an IVP showed a mass 1-2 cm in size arising in the middle of his right ureter. His urologist had recommended a right nephrectomy. He and mother were planning to visit me at Duke. I urged him to bring the IVP. He felt well. I arranged for him to see the chief of urology, Dr. David Paulson, who suggested he could perform a more limited surgical procedure, remove the tumor, and spare the kidney. Dad had his surgery at Duke within a week. We did not know the pathology but feared it would be a carcinoma. I'll never forget the way the urology resident said to me in the recovery room, as he was wheeling Dad out of the OR, with all the empathy of a bulldozer, "yeah, it's a cancer all right, a big one." The tumor was several centimeters in diameter. It had penetrated the muscularis of the ureter. Several periureteral nodes were positive. Dad recovered from his surgery in about one week and was discharged to my apartment. We listened to one of his favorite pieces of music, the New World Symphony, embraced and cried because his training and mine told us what the likely outcome of this diagnosis would be. I knew, from burrowing into the epidemiology of transitional cell carcinoma of the ureter, that the five-year survival rate was less than 5 percent. Dad did not ask me to obtain articles about the disease. He played the role of patient rather well. He did not challenge his physicians. He did not ask many questions. He knew, in fall 1979, he would probably not be alive in five years.

Marriage

The most important decision I ever made was to say hello to Paula Thomas, RN, on the Cardiology Ward of Duke Hospital-South, before Duke Hospital-North opened. Late on the evening of March 15, 1979, she stood transferring orders before she went off duty at Duke for the last time. She had learned a few days earlier that her father, a general surgeon, was suffering with small cell carcinoma of the lung, and she would return to her home in Texas in two days to help her mother, a nurse, care for him. Of course, I did not know any of this. I saw a beautiful nurse with a wonderful smile. I was trying to get home after a long night on duty, but I stopped to talk with her. She recalls that she spoke first. I must have noticed immediately, although I did not understand its significance until much later, that she could love someone unconditionally. I learned she was leaving in two days. I offered to take her to dinner the next night. We went out two nights in a row, and we kept in touch long distance. I proposed to her that summer while she visited me and my family in Washington, D.C. She accepted. We married March 15, 1980, while her father and mine were in remission and feeling well. We left our wedding reception and drove all the next two days in her car, towing a U-HAUL trailer, to return to Duke where I had clinic on March 18. I recall saying to Paula before we married that I did not know what I would do for a living, but I did not think I would practice medicine full time. She wanted to marry a physician like her father, but she told me to follow my interests. She trusted my judgment. Eighteen months later, our first child was born. We named him James, after her father.

Robert Wood Johnson Clinical Scholar

After I completed my residency in Internal Medicine in June 1981, I increased my commute slightly by driving to the medical center of the University of North Carolina, Chapel Hill, from our apartment in Durham. My wife and I bought our first home in Chapel Hill just after I completed residency. That was the first and last dwelling I owned or rented that did not contain at least one personal computer. At UNC I learned about variations in medical practice around the nation. I heard about John Wennberg, MD and his small area variation studies. I met biostatisticians and epidemiologists intrigued with measuring the outcomes of care and with risk-adjusting for patients' characteristics to compare the effectiveness of treatment. I learned basic medical economics.

As a Robert Wood Johnson Scholar, I studied with two consummate general internists, Bob and Suzanne Fletcher, husband and wife, who had met as class-mates at Harvard Medical School a few years before I studied there. They encour-aged me to enroll in a degree program at UNC, and I chose the Master of Public Health degree, concentrating in epidemiology and thinking that I would be better prepared for life as an academic neurologist if I had such training. But, in my heart of hearts, I knew that I would not return to full-time clinical practice, even though I excelled at it at Duke, and enjoyed it. I wanted to learn about patterns of treat-ment and variations in medical care and why physicians, hospitals, and the "medi-cal-industrial complex" were so focused on high-technology treatments of diseases, most of which could have been avoided. I discovered that the computer held the answer to many such questions because it could complete the mathematical anal-ysis of patterns in data so much faster than people with slide rules and calculators.

In the basement of the School of Public Health of UNC, guarded by a priesthood of computer operators and systems analysts, stood a large blue computer from IBM that processed the statistical equations and data I relied on to complete homework in epidemiology and biostatistics. I had to wait days for the results of each run to return to me. Usually, a simple typographical error or faulty syntax in computer grammar led the computer to reject my work without processing. When it did accept the programs and data, it usually did not produce analyses that answered all my questions, but I had to see the results before I would recognize that I needed to do still more analyses. The time it took me to produce homework irritated me, but I had no alternatives at the time. All graduate students labored over keypunch machines making cards; trudged to the basement of the building; entered a queue; filled out job request forms; entered another queue; submitted punched cards that they had not folded, spindled, or mutilated to a slightly snide operator; and prayed for hours or days their jobs would run this time. This was in 1981, not so long ago, and more than seven years after the Altair 8800 personal computer kit went on sale from MITS in Albuquerque, after Apple incorporated to sell Apple II's, after Radio Shack began selling the TRS-80, but before IBM gave birth to the PC.

In late 1981, I began working with several members of the faculty on a project that became the basis of my master's thesis in epidemiology. We had access to a mini-computer in the School of Public Health that gave users a monitor and a keyboard for an interface. The monitor took up less room than the IBM monitors on the patient care units of Duke North Hospital, from which I obtained the results of lab-oratory tests performed on my patients, but it allowed me and my co-authors to interact with the computer and test statistical analyses immediately. We were using a time-sharing system that supported multiple simultaneous users. I never returned to the punched cards and never regretted their absence from my work. I had to ana-lyze data originally collected for a study by the Centers for Disease Control of noso-comial infections in community hospitals in the United States. In the data set of dis-charge abstract information on inpatients, we knew who owned each hospital and whether it was for-profit, private not-for-profit, or public not-for-profit. We wanted to know why hospitals in the East kept patients an average of about three days longer than hospitals in the West, and what proportion of the variation in length of stay of those patients could be explained by the ownership of the hospitals in which they received treatment.

We created a risk-adjustment methodology using length of stay as the dependent variable and using diagnosis codes and demographic factors of patients as predictors (independent variables) of length of stay. We explained about one-half the variation in length of stay. We could not explain more than about one-third of the regional variation in length of stay with our regression equation. We discovered that for-profit hospitals kept patients several days more than predicted by the risk-adjustment model we developed.

I finished my class work for the master's degree in one year. I held a two-year fellowship from the Robert Wood Johnson foundation and did not want to stay at UNC and continue to work as a general medicine fellow, performing preoperative assessments of patients for the surgeons, for a second year. Health care economics fascinated me. The entrepreneurial ferment in health care, coinciding with the advent of managed care, beckoned to me. I wanted to know if I could take some of the tenets of health promotion, disease prevention, and epidemiology and use them to build a company, or companies, that would substantially improve the health and welfare of Americans. I wanted to know if I could use the insights gleaned from working with large databases of patients' demographic and clinical data to teach physicians about the large variation that exists in their habits of practice. How could we explain the large differences in length of stay among patients on the East Coast and the West Coast and between for-profit and not-for-profit hospitals? I did not want to stay in the abstract, theoretical world of academics. I realized that I wanted to make a difference in the world of patient care, health plans, and health care technology.

So, I interviewed at the graduate schools of business at UNC and Duke to ask them about opportunities for me to study health care economics and management with them. Both suggested that I study at a school with faculty expert in health care finance and management. Remember, these interviews took place in spring 1982, before the business schools of Duke and UNC had invested in building their expertise in the health care industry. The deans of those schools suggested I study at Stanford, because Stanford had two of the most influential health care economists in Alain Enthoven and Victor Fuchs. I approached the leaders of the Robert Wood Johnson Foundation who supervised the RWJ Fellowship programs, and I talked with Suzanne and Bob Fletcher, the co-directors of my program, about the possibility of transferring my fellowship to Stanford. They said they would let me transfer if I were accepted to the program. The dean of admission of Stanford's business school called me personally to invite me to attend the school. They were pleased to have a physician in the class. Only a few other Robert Wood Johnson Clinical Scholars had taken an MBA at Stanford. It was nice to feel needed.

Studies at Stanford

When I applied to Stanford, I thought that graduate business school would be like the school of public health. My expectations proved wrong. The Graduate School of

Business (GSB) overwhelmed me with work and undermined my sense of peace by confronting me with the specter that I was wasting two valuable years of my life. I had to learn financial accounting and found the subject less intuitive, and more difficult to master, than neuroanatomy had been in medical school. The first semester of the first year of business school held many dark days for me. Of the nearly 400 students in my class, all but sixty were younger than I was. I celebrated my 30th birthday in fall of that first year. With no business, accounting, or marketing experience to rely on, every subject was new to me. I made another mistake. I had taken biostatistics at the School of Public Health at UNC. I had a choice of taking statistics for first-year students or advanced statistics. I took advanced statistics. I learned later that students with master's degrees in statistics took the basic course in order to have more time for the new material. I was taking advanced statistics from a graduate student new to the United States from Bombay, or Calcutta, or New Delhi, with an accent so thick I could barely understand him and no tolerance for anyone who could not perform Fourier analyses in his sleep. On weekends, I worked for 24 or 36 hours in the emergency department of the Palo Alto Veterans Hospital to earn extra money for our small family. I had friends learning to perform lucrative procedures in fellowships in cardiology and gastroenterology, and there I was learning financial accounting and advanced statistics as a basic student again. Paula felt depressed that I spent so little time at home, staying up late working on homework assignments in the computer center in the basement of the GSB. All in all, the first semester undermined my sense of self and my resolve to complete business school.

There was one other physician in my class. Someone who had just completed a general surgery residency at Peter Bent Brigham Hospital (it had not yet merged with Women's Hospital) decided he could make a fortune in venture capital. He lasted as long as the first mid-term exam in financial accounting, about two months into the school year. The average grade was about a 45 on a scale of 100 points. A number of the CPAs in the class who had failed the exemption exam for the financial accounting course said it was the hardest accounting test they had ever taken. I scored a 26, and felt utterly disconsolate. I was squandering my youth, I told myself while bicycling home at the end of that day, studying business. I should be out practicing medicine, I told myself. The general surgeon did not return to class after that test. I learned later he had taken a cardiac surgery fellowship at the University of Arkansas. He would be making much more money than I would be making, I knew. I did not enjoy surgery. I did not envy him, but he was using his clinical skills and I was letting mine atrophy. The work at the VA hospital gave me some practice, but not enough to keep me as sharp in internal medicine as I had been at Duke and Chapel Hill. But I plugged on.

The second semester improved my spirits considerably. I took an elective from Alain Enthoven in health care economics. I took the first of several marketing classes. I loved health care economics, and I loved marketing. A small and, for me, uninteresting part of marketing is advertising. The much larger and more interesting aspect of marketing involves strategic planning and figuring out who your customers are and what they want. I thought medicine spent too much time deciding what patients needed, including, it seemed to me, ever more expensive and invasive diagnostic and therapeutic measures. By the end of the first year, I knew that I wanted to complete the second year and looked forward to the electives I could take.

My classmates were as bright as they were in Harvard Medical School but entirely different in demeanor. In medical school, we learned from lecturers, lecture notes, and text books. We spent relatively little time learning from each other. We dissected cadavers as teams, but we learned independently, each bringing to the study of the cadaver and the human body his or her own intensity and curiosity. We studied long hours. We worked in teams in clinical rotations, but learning came from senior house officers, fellows, and attendings more than from fellow students. We studied medical cases on rounds in groups, but we did not work up the patients in groups. Each student took his or her own patients. We led relatively isolated lives in medical school. We spent very little time producing reports or presentations as a team. We were the best and the brightest of medical students, our faculty told us, but we were loners, accustomed to long hours hitting the books to memorize a mammoth mountain of facts. In medical school, if fellow students came to class unprepared, I was not the worse for it. I did not even know. We listened to a lecturer and took notes torridly. My learning did not depend on how well other students prepared for class. Business school could not have been more different.

Stanford's Graduate School of Business depends heavily on the case method of education. We read books and took courses such as financial accounting and statistics, with heavy doses of homework prepared by each individual student, but after the basic science courses of the first semester, the curriculum emphasized case courses. Class discussion taught the material, and lecturers facilitated lively discussion among the students, whose observations taught the class various ways of considering business situations. When other students were not prepared, I suffered, because I could not learn from their insights. When I came unprepared, they suffered.

My classmates at Stanford Business School were far less introverted than those at Harvard Medical School. These students were eager for class discussion and thrived on an active social life after class. Married, a physician at heart, naturally shy, tending to introspection and self-doubt, I did not mix much with students after class. I worked at the VA hospital often. I did not feel an integral part of the class. I felt decidedly different from most of the students, who were still dating, still in their early twenties, and still completely unfamiliar with the health care system. Most of them wondered why someone who had completed a residency in medicine and a master of public health would want a business degree. The time was the early 1980s, and managed care received attention in the press, but most physicians still earned far more prestige and income than 99 percent of business executives. I thought the world was going to change, and thought knowledge of business matters would help me manage the care of populations of people over time. I did not understand that our lives change more slowly than the purveyors of change, the writers and the pundits, incessantly predict.

I found fascinating the intellectual debates about costs and benefits of business decisions, marketing strategies, and issues of information systems planning. I took an elective information systems planning course in the business and learned that minicomputers were replacing mainframes for much work. The personal computer did not have much significance then, in 1983. The IBM PC had been released the year before, and it could not do much. The business of linking personal computers with local area networks had not begun to blossom. No one knew about the future advent of the World Wide Web or about standardized corporate intranets.

I studied medical informatics at Stanford's School of Medicine, in a class taught by my former intern, Ted Shortliffe, MD, PhD, now an assistant professor of medicine and computer science at Stanford. We talked about databases but little about relational databases, because they were so new. No one had yet heard of object databases. I enjoyed the courses in medical informatics and saw what I believed to be an important future role for information systems in helping physicians and managers manage demand for health care services.

In spring of my first year, I became thoroughly disenchanted with the computer laboratory at the Graduate School of Business. I needed to use a computer for a number of classes, and the computer lab included about 30 dumb terminals connected to a DEC minicomputer. We had text screens, no menus, no point-and-click graphical user interface. We did simple calculations with calculators. We created and calculated sophisticated equations in the computer lab. We played Space Invaders in our spare time. I was amazed at how much better an interactive session with a computer monitor and keyboard was than the teletype I had used in high school or the stacks of punch cards I used at Chapel Hill in the School of Public Health. I could interact directly with the computer and enter data and produce results. I liked those features. But I did not like having to wait in line for a terminal or working late in the computer lab.

So, in early 1983, I bought my first personal computer. I considered the IBM PC but found it dull. The Macintosh had not come out, and the Apple II looked like a toy, with large fonts and little to see on the screen. I noticed that Texas Instruments and Digital Equipment Corporation had both improved on the original IBM PC design, using video standards with higher resolution and more colors than the IBM PC. I did not understand at the time that software vendors found those competing standards an expensive nuisance, because they had to write their software drivers for either IBM, or DEC, or TI, or all three. I bought a TI Professional PC, with the TI versions of MS-DOS, Microsoft Multiplan and Wordstar. Now I could write reports, perform financial analyses, and prepare graphs and charts without using the computer center. I never went back and did not miss it. I spent about $5,000 for a TI 300 dpi dot matrix printer, TI Professional PC with 8086 processor, 256K of RAM, and two floppy disk drives. Many students visited our apartment to see this digital wonder. We all agreed that the TI had graphics superior to the IBM PC. Little did I know that the TI standard would not create enough of a market and that TI would drop its standard in favor of the IBM compatible CGA standard within two years.

Not long after I bought the TI Professional PC, I installed a 10 MB hard disk for which I paid $1,000 that I had earned at the VA. I installed another 512K of RAM memory for about $1,000, not knowing that DOS only addressed 640K. I hope the computer store clerks did not know this either, but they probably did, taking advantage of my naiveté about personal computers. Still, I loved the system. It freed me from the computer center and gave me a spreadsheet program, Multiplan, with much better graphics than the DEC financial planning software and dumb terminals in the computer center. Thinking back, I am amazed at what I can do today. I was amazed then at what I could do with a PC.

I used Multiplan for about one year, until I read about and saw Lotus 123. The speed of processing (it was written in Assembler to maximize speed) and the graphics awed me. I bought the version for the TI Professional as soon as I could. I never missed Multiplan, and Microsoft took more than 10 years to take the lead again in spreadsheets for PCs, with Microsoft Excel 7.0 for Windows 95.

After the first year, we were encouraged to take a summer internship in a business. I chose to work for Kaiser-Permanente Health Plan in its primary care internal medicine clinic one day each week and in the Economics and Planning Office for the Northern California region four days a week. I enjoyed a chance to work for Bruce Sams, MD, a cardiologist and the head of the Permanente Medical Group in Northern California, and Barney Rhodes, MD, a dermatologist and the senior physician in the corporate offices of Kaiser-Permanente. In the Economics and Planning Office, I took the assignment to develop a risk-adjustment method to calculate expected use of nursing hours per patient stay, and per patient day, for the 13 hospitals Kaiser-Permanente then operated in Northern California. We built a risk-adjustment method for nursing hours per patient day and nursing hours per patient stay and then calculated expected use of nursing time for each patient care unit of each hospital. We confirmed what senior management had expected, that budgeting for nursing took place with different rules at each facility.

What impressed me most in the study were the analytical resources I had at my disposal. We studied data from hundreds of thousands of inpatients over multiple years, stored in the Statistical Analysis System in a mainframe devoted to analytical work. I could call on analysts with doctorates in statistics to help me formulate my queries. I used an IBM 3270 terminal and JCL and SAS to do my work. I knew the fee-for-service community had nothing like the discipline and analytical firepower I found in Kaiser. I suspected they would have a hard time competing with this well-informed medical juggernaut.

During an occasional lunch with Dr. Sams, or Dr. Rhodes, or both, I heard how important they thought it was to train physicians in health care management. They faced multimillion to multibillion dollar management decisions frequently. They encouraged me to continue my studies. I returned to Stanford in the fall, convinced that I had chosen the right field of medicine—organizational medicine—in which to specialize. I also returned convinced that computers would play a key role in the analysis of practice habits of clinicians and would lead to more standardized and higher quality care.

I do not recall all the courses I took in my second year of business school, but I remember the ones I loved, specifically two courses in entrepreneurship taught by Steven Brandt, who wrote the popular book *Ten Steps to Entrepreneurship*, and one in observational astronomy. Steven Brandt's courses showed me how exciting and rewarding, emotionally and financially, starting one's own business could be. I charged into study of every case we considered. I participated actively in the class discussions. I could not get enough of strategic planning and market research. As a wonderful counterpoint to such close attention to the details of small businesses, I loved a graduate course in astronomy offered in the Graduate School of Arts and Sciences that taught me how to photograph the moons of Jupiter, how to measure the height of mountains on the Moon, and how to interpret the nuclear equations explaining the production of heavier elements from hydrogen in the nuclear furnaces of stars.

Perhaps the most profoundly moving lesson I learned at Stanford came from that astronomy class, when I realized that every atom in me, every heavy atom in the earth, was created billions of years ago in the center of a star long since exploded and no longer visible. The vast scope of the known universe overwhelmed me and served as a useful balance to the intricacies of business management. My fellow students in astronomy, with whom I spent many a long, cold night shivering in the Stanford observatory exposing film to the faint light from a distant planet, star, or galaxy, could not fathom why a trained physician would be studying a marketing case while waiting to develop a photograph of a lunar mountain range. I could only say that I wanted to learn about medicine, business, and astronomy. I enjoy learning. I enjoy the role of student. I wish I could continue that role forever. But I knew I had to pay for a home and the education of my children and save money.

One of the most frustrating experiences of business school involved a medical center. For one of the courses on entrepreneurship, students had to produce a strategic plan for an existing firm whose business was changing. Two classmates and I selected the Palo Alto Clinic, a multispecialty group practice of more than 200 physicians located close to Stanford. I knew Palo Alto Clinic's excellent reputation for clinical work. Most physicians had admitting privileges and teaching roles at Stanford University Medical Center. The year was 1984. Managed care had entered the Bay Area, with IPAs forming up and down the San Francisco Peninsula. Palo Alto Clinic looked like most other large multispecialty groups at the time, heavily dominated by procedural and subspecialist physicians. My two classmates had no clinical training, but each considered business consulting to the health care industry a likely career. We interviewed the leaders, heard about the management issues and studied information systems and market data and trends in health insurance and managed care.

We learned that each physician depended on his or her billed charges ("productivity") for income. The Clinic paid few physicians any money for administrative work. Little attention or planning went into business planning. The Clinic appeared well-organized only from the outside of its principal building. From the inside, the Palo Alto Clinic of 1984 behaved more like a collection of independent practices sharing office space and some administrative services than a disciplined business capable of drafting and executing a strategic plan. The Clinic had antiquated information systems. It retained very little of its income for future growth and distributed most of its profits to partners. It funded capital investments through cash flow.

We looked at Kaiser's growth and considered the substantial resources for data analysis and business planning at the disposal of its leaders. We noted the growth of independent practice associations and other health plans that would steer patients away from the Palo Alto Clinic. We observed large numbers of subspecialists living and working in and around Palo Alto. We wrote a plan filled with strategic threats and opportunities. It called for change in governance and in organization of priorities and for discipline in retention and allocation of capital. We urged the group to give up its model of every-man-for-himself earnings and financial management and to retain capital for expansion of plant and equipment, especially information systems, and for development of a primary care network of providers and an insurance product. I learned later that our strategic plan, for which the Palo Alto Clinic paid nothing except the time of a few senior executives to meet with us, did not appeal to those leaders. I also know that the Clinic, and other clinics like it across the nation, in the succeeding decade paid hundreds of thousands of dollars to consulting firms for unflattering competitive analyses and strategic plans such as we gave the Palo Alto Clinic for free. As a consolation, our professor gave us a high mark for our work. My interest and belief in the enormous potential competitive advantage of multispecialty group practice as an organization of medical expertise and resources dates from my study of the Palo Alto Clinic.

Paula was pregnant with our second child in early 1984, during my last semester of business school. My father had developed metastases to his thoracic vertebra of transitional cell carcinoma of the ureter originally resected at Duke while I was an intern. In the fourth year after his surgery, he developed back pain and a lytic lesion in one of his lower thoracic vertebra, which was treated with irradiation. Our second son, who would be named Marshall, after me and my Dad, was due to be born in early June 1984. My father began losing weight in March and complained of constant abdominal pain made worse by eating. He lost his appetite. His weight plummeted from a portly 220 pounds to about 170. Physical examinations and CT scans revealed no tumor bulk in his abdomen. I flew from San Francisco to Washington several times in the last months of his life and the last months of my term at Stanford. I implored him to eat and tried to convince him, a psychiatrist who taught psychosomatic medicine to medical students and residents at George Washington University, that his anorexia must be psychological. Why else would CT and MRI scans not show tumor bulk. He had no detectable ascites. Those days were rough, losing a parent, finishing graduate school and preparing for the arrival of our second child all at once.

During spring 1984, from across the country, I heard of Dad's miserable experience with the health care system, visiting various specialists in various locations without anyone acting in charge, having medical records lost, repeating tests, being made sick with radiation therapy. Everyone was excessively optimistic about his chances, but no one took responsibility for his total care. What my Dad needed was a doctor, to paraphrase Eugene Stead, MD, the legendary chief of medicine at Duke. As his only son, I felt more than guilty studying business in California.

Gaining a Son, Losing My Father

In May, Dad became too weak to eat. He was admitted to Georgetown University Hospital for diagnostic evaluation by his chosen internist. Our second son, Marshall, was born on June 7. I finished my term projects and course examinations and shipped our belongings to Florida, where I had accepted the job of Medical Director for the Watson Clinic in Lakeland. I cried with Dad before he died. I begged him to eat and to stay well while I tried to get on my feet in my chosen career of medical management. I worried that he would not approve of my choices. He said he did. He said that medicine was changing and that he thought my interest in epidemiology, informatics, and management would pay off for me.

In the hospital, we learned he had a smoldering disseminated intravascular coagulation. He looked like a neglected prisoner of war, so gaunt and haggard. I had seen that appearance of metastatic carcinoma on hundreds of patients, but I refused to see it on him. I clung to a conviction that all he needed to do was change his attitude, and he would start to eat and return to his family. He suffered a brainstem infarction one morning in late May, while I was in Washington from California to check on him. I walked into his room, said "Hi, Dad," and noticed his disconjugate gaze. Out of a stupor, he said, "Hi, Marsh," and did not say much else to me ever again.

I had completed internal medicine training with a year of neurology and had seen many patients in many hospitals in North Carolina, Virginia, and California begin to plummet downhill, just like Dad. I barked orders and became my father's internist.

We moved Dad to the ICU. He suffered another brainstem infarction, slipped into a coma, his DIC worsened, and I saw that he was not going to recover. He became decerebrate and showed no signs of recovery after 10 days. His general internist, a semi-retired dandy with whom my father played golf occasionally, talked to me and my mother in a patronizing way about placing a feeding gastrostomy and shipping Dad to a nursing home. I knew Dad would want no part of that plan. I conferred with my mother and sister, and I told the physician we wanted Dad kept comfortable, without surgery. We moved him back to a medical floor. I removed his IV and NG tube. He was not on a ventilator. He died quietly a week later, in hospital, on June 21, 1984. At autopsy he had disseminated peritoneal carcinomatosis. No wonder he could not eat.

The Watson Clinic

My wife, two children, and I moved to Lakeland, Florida, where I worked for the Watson Clinic as a general internist one-half of my time and as the Medical Director the other half. I was recruited to bring some business planning to the group of 75 physicians, all trained in the United States and all board-certified in their specialties. My experience with the Palo Alto Clinic led me to believe that multispecialty group practice had far better strategic business opportunities than hospitals. I turned down a job as Medical Director of a large hospital in Washington, D.C., in order to work for the Watson Clinic.

To indicate the importance given to the role of Medical Director, I was the youngest physician in the group and had to wait two years of probationary training to become a partner, yet I had responsibility for handling all complaints by patients about physicians. I attended all meetings of the Executive Committee ex officio. Soon I became involved in planning for a new practice management system and led the procurement committee. The procurement helped me understand the importance of defining requirements before considering vendors. Vendors want to show you the shiniest features of their systems, and those shiny features may dazzle you. If you forget to list all the reasons you need a computer system and all the functions you expect it to perform, you may forget them and select the shiniest system that, only after implementation, you discover cannot perform certain functions necessary to the operation of your group.

Not long after arriving, I made a point of meeting all the clinicians and administrative personnel in the Watson Clinic. One person with a senior position in finance spent most of her time calculating manually the distribution of income among partners. The formula for partners was simple, but the calculations were iterative and extraordinarily time-consuming. Partners received their income after all expenses of the clinic were paid, including salaries to employed physicians. The formula dictated that 5 percent of income be distributed by seniority, with 1 percent per year, to a maximum of 5 years, given to each physician after partnership. Twenty-five percent was distributed equally to all partners and served to transfer income from procedural physicians to primary care physicians. The remainder, 70 percent of available funds, was shared in proportion to each physician's productivity, defined as each physician's proportion of billed charges divided by the total of all partners' billed charges.

I decided that I would create a spreadsheet program to calculate partners' distribution of income. I used Lotus 123, and spent several evenings building the financial model. It worked and saved the accountant, who had never worked with a personal computer before, countless hours. She received my gift as a mixed blessing. She trusted her calculations. She worried that the computer would make a mistake. But, after spending days testing the numbers produced in seconds by the computer, she could see her time was better spent on other work for the Clinic. I sold my TI Professional PC to the Clinic to automate her work, and I bought another computer from Texas Instruments, a portable with a small color screen that used standard IBM EGA graphics. It had 640K of RAM, an 80286 processor and a 20 MB hard disk built into its 30-pound case.

In the hospital and clinics, I saw patients with chronic medical complaints, including diabetes, hypertension, asthma, angina, chronic obstructive pulmonary disease, and cirrhosis. I thoroughly enjoyed working with the excellent clinicians of the Clinic. Having every specialty available on call every night and weekend gave me great comfort. Partners covered partners closely and helped whenever they could. I enjoyed practice at the Clinic more than at any other place I had worked, including Harvard, Duke, Chapel Hill, countless emergency departments in North Carolina and Virginia where I moonlighted for extra money, the Palo Alto VA, and Kaiser-Permanente clinics. But I wanted to know more about management and computers. I believed our society would have to restructure medicine to continue to afford it and to emphasize prevention and primary care over high-tech diagnosis and treatment of preventable diseases.

Jack Whitehead, the builder of Technicon into a multi-million dollar manufacturer of automated blood analysis machines for clinical laboratories (the SMAC analyzers) and purveyor of other hospital supplies, sold Technicon to Revlon in the early 1980s. He wanted to use some of the $400,000,000 he earned from its sale to finance the creation of a national network of HMOs affiliated with multispecialty group practices. He flew into Lakeland on his personal jet to woo the leaders of the Watson Clinic to join his national network of multispecialty group practices, that he said already included the Cleveland Clinic, Scott & White, Palo Alto Clinic, and Geisinger Clinic, among others. Never mind that several of the Clinics already owned HMOs; the idea of a national HMO based on an organized network of well-regarded provider organizations appealed to me. At the time, I had begun to feel stifled at the Watson Clinic. The partners did not want any more central control and discipline in the clinic than the partners of the Palo Alto Clinic wanted in theirs. I worried about the long-term success of the Watson Clinic and about my ability to grow personally and professionally in an organization whose owners did not really value medical executives.

I offered to work with Jack Whitehead on the business plan for the project if the Watson Clinic joined. I mentioned my training at Stanford. He knew some of my professors at Stanford. He finished his presentation, climbed in his jet, and flew off. The Watson Clinic partners eventually voted to join the organization Whitehead was forming. Nevertheless, the other clinics quarreled with Whitehead over control of the organization, and the venture collapsed. Whitehead had agreed to put up two-thirds of the capital for one-third of the equity in the new venture, but the clinic leaders thought he was still getting too much ownership. They thought they could do the work themselves. Whitehead quit in disgust. I did not expect to hear from him again.

To my surprise, about three months later, he called me asking if I would leave Watson Clinic to help him create a national network of HMOs affiliated with academic medical centers. This time, he told me, he would retain control of the management company that managed these HMOs, and he wanted me to be the Vice President and Medical Director of that company. We would use the successful model of Tufts Affiliated Health Plan, and the executive who had built Tufts into a large and profitable HMO, Allen Reilly, had already agreed to join this new venture as President. With Jack's money and contacts, Allen's expertise, and my education and energy, we could not lose. Jack and I agreed. I did talk about the venture with Jerry Grossman, MD, then President of New England Medical Center, who suggested that the world did not need another HMO development company and that the success of TAHP might not translate to other locations. He was probably trying to tell me to watch out for Jack and Allen, but I did not hear him. I wanted to leave the Watson Clinic and Lakeland. Six months before we left, Paula gave birth to our third son, Christopher, and I knew I wanted to raise my children in a more cosmopolitan area than Lakeland, Florida.

University Health Partners

I ignored an omen when I met Allen Reilly for our first interview in a hotel in Tampa, Florida, just after dusk and a violent thunderstorm. The hotel was completely blacked out, so we talked in the dark. I could not have recognized him later by sight if my life had depended on it. I only knew his voice. Nevertheless, his plans were ambitious, and I wanted to exercise my entrepreneurial talents. Jack and Allen agreed with my conviction that we would have to have information systems that were second to none and standardize them across the nation to produce a national database for retrospective analysis for quality improvement and outcomes studies. They also agreed to locate the corporate offices of University Health Partners (UHP) in northern Virginia, near my home in Washington, D.C. I accepted their offer. I would earn a salary comparable to what I made at Watson Clinic and would vest in 5 percent of the company stock over five years. Allen suggested I accept a six-month severance package in case things went badly. It had not occurred to me to ask for a severance package. I announced that I would leave the Watson Clinic exactly two weeks after I had been elected partner, in March 1986. To earn partnership, an employed physician had to have 90 percent of the partners voting for him. The vote on me was close, but my supporters prevailed.

UHP never was profitable and lasted only about 18 months. Jack Whitehead, then in his mid-sixties, enjoyed jetting from academic center to academic center enticing senior management to joint venture HMOs with the firm. He conceived of the company with Paul Ellwood, MD, who brought Jack in to help the University of Minnesota decide what to do with its new university hospital that had no patients in it because it had no contracts with payers. Jack used his capital to purchase a failing primary care HMO with fewer than 10,000 covered lives, renamed the health plan Health Partners, and Health Partners began advertising that it had an exclusive contract with the University of Minnesota Medical Center. Taking a new HMO to the Twin Cities of Minnesota in spring 1986 was worse than taking coal to Newcastle. Still, the marketing appeal worked, though not in the way Jack had intended. All the other HMOs in the Twin Cities contracted with the University Hospital so they would not be left out. Health Partners struggled to survive, but could not make much headway in such a managed care intensive market.

Meanwhile, Jack, Allen Reilly, and I went on the road to promote our model of university health plans. We interested Duke and the University of Virginia, both institutions well known to Jack and to me.

I learned a painful but valuable lesson with UHP. Most people, and especially those in academic health centers, do not like to say no to you if they can avoid it. They kill you with indecision, procrastination, and countless committee meetings. The sales cycle takes forever. At Duke and UVA, leaders wanted to keep on the good side of Jack Whitehead. He had endowed the Whitehead Institute at MIT with about $100,000,000 and promised a gift to Duke of $10,000,000. We were proposing a radical design for a health plan. We wanted our health plans to distinguish themselves in the market for their quality of care. We wanted to screen potential physicians with quality indicators and exclude from our panels of physicians as many as one-half the practitioners in areas surrounding our partner academic centers. We wanted our plans to have a reputation for selectivity at a time when most HMOs contracted with anyone that accepted their low fee schedules. We naively thought that selectivity would appeal to these medical centers. It did not, but they did not tell us so until we had consumed millions of dollars in legal and actuarial fees working with them to design our joint ventures. The medical centers we chose to work with first wanted no part of excluding any potential referring physician. They wanted no chance that a referring physician would become angry with them and send fee-for-service referrals elsewhere. While academicians and their house officers speak condescendingly about LMDs (local medical doctors) who refer patients to them, they do not want to reduce the flow of those referrals in any way.

To make a long story short, we spent nine months trying to give birth to an HMO at Duke and were given promising reports at every meeting with senior management, until the final faculty vote went against us. We were told Duke did not want to participate in an HMO in 1987. After nearly a year at the University of Virginia, our champion, the Chancellor of the Medical Center, announced his retirement, and the new Chancellor, who had not yet arrived on the scene, sent word that he wanted to postpone the decision to create an HMO until he arrived and could assess the market for an HMO in central Virginia.

Jack White had had enough. He had never faced the obfuscation, delays, and dissembling he faced in trying to lead academic medical centers to make a commitment to a business venture. We had the right talent. We had the right experience. We had Jack's considerable money. We could have kept going, but Jack was fed up. We decided in June 1987 to fold our tent on July 1. I had six months to find a job. Our fourth son, Sterling, had arrived in April 1987, and I worried about finding a job with enough security and income that I could raise our four sons and provide for them the extraordinary educational opportunities that I had had.

In retrospect, for all our experience with HMOs and universities, we were incredibly naïve and overly optimistic. We were not wrong in our vision, but in our timing. Now, 10 years later, Duke and UVA have HMOs that are central to their strategic plans to remain competitive referral centers for their regions. The University of Minnesota Medical Center has not fared as well.

Inter+Net Health System and Inova Health System

After UHP, finding a job did not prove difficult. I contacted the President of Inova Health System, Knox Singleton, and described my education, background, and interests. He offered me the new position of Senior Vice President of Inter+Net Health System, a PPO of 13 hospitals in greater Washington that Inova was organizing in joint venture with Georgetown University Medical Center. Inova was then, in fall 1987, a new name for the Fairfax Hospital System of four hospitals in Fairfax County, Virginia, across the Potomac River from Washington, D.C. Fairfax Hospital, the flagship tertiary care center of Inova, serves as a secondary teaching hospital for Georgetown, and many physicians who trained at Georgetown establish practices in Fairfax, or they did until the population growth moved 10 miles farther west. Inter+Net (the name was Internet until we discovered that a little known academic and research-oriented telecommunication network was called the Internet) was meant to help member hospitals compete with the more than 26 other hospitals in greater Washington. Staff members of Inter+Net were employees of Inova Health System who were leased to Inter+Net to get it going.

Inter+Net started as most regional associations of hospitals do, as a purchasing organization. The CEOs of the hospitals made up the board of directors. A hospital administrator who helped establish a PPO in Arkansas was recruited to serve as the President of Inter+Net. We started trying to build a shared laundry, establish a shared health plan for hospital employees that would grow into a regional health plan (staff members were told not to use the word HMO), and negotiate purchasing contracts with regional suppliers. I saw the importance of a regional data warehouse for systematic quality improvement studies, outcomes management, and health services research. I recalled the power of such technology I saw Kaiser use. I tried to generate enthusiasm for a shared communications network. I argued that the hospitals could share a marketing program based on a nurse advice line.

I was woefully, naively sanguine about the wisdom of my ideas. I did not anticipate the provincial opposition I would face from departmental managers whose incentives heavily favored their own departments over the success of shared services sponsored by Inter+Net. Even hospital executives who sat on the board of Inter+Net told their staffs to do whatever was best for their hospital, and support Inter+Net when it was convenient.

We did launch the nurse advice line, over the explicit objections of the marketing directors of the hospitals, who did not want to see money allocated for their departments diverted to promotion of Inter+Net. We convinced the board of directors of Inter+Net that such a service would generate valuable goodwill in the community and lead to referrals to hospital services and physicians affiliated with their facilities. The goodwill they felt good about. The referrals they cared about. We argued that we could develop the service ourselves, but the directors wanted us to contract with an established service. On looking, we found Ask-A-Nurse and contracted with what was then called Referral Systems Group, a small firm spun off of the Adventist Health West hospital network. We contracted with them for nursing protocols, training, and software.

We hired 30 nurses, trained them, set up 16 nurses' stations with computer monitors to our database of triage instructions, and began taking calls. We saved several lives, one from an insulin-induced coma and one from meningitis, by alerting family members to take patients to emergency departments when they would have left them alone to sleep off their illnesses. Our nurses and I, the medical director, were on local news broadcasts several times. We answered more than 1,000 telephone calls a day and made numerous referrals. But the marketing directors whined that our referral program, because it employed expensive nurses and gave advice without referrals to about 40 percent of callers, was too expensive, and that their programs—and each was planning to start his or her own—would be more cost effective for them.

The hospital CIOs dutifully attended meetings we called and spoke in glowing terms about the benefits of standardization of networks, applications, and data dictionaries among the participating institutions. Then they went back to their facilities and ignored the discussions. Not one had the courage to promote standardization if such standardization meant increasing his budget. Each wanted to manage a departmental budget. None wanted to champion a shared program that might cost his organization more money in standardization in the short run. The hospital executives did not understand the issues of standardization or the benefits of a shared data repository for clinical care and retrospective quality improvement studies. In information systems planning, nothing happened.

Then the marketplace for managed care became very competitive, and payers refused to deal with Inter+Net, which they saw as an elaborate boycott. They gave better deals to hospitals outside of Inter+Net than through it, and support for Inter+Net began to crumble. Inter+Net began its slow collapse in about 1990 and ceased to exist in about 1993. There went my dreams of a standardized electronic network, standardized clinical applications shared by all the hospitals, and a standardized nursing triage for the metropolitan Washington area. We tried to do all these programs in a predominantly fee-for-service medical economy through an organization without much internal stability.

Three years later, the marketing director of Inova, who in meetings of Inter+Net marketing directors supported the Ask-A-Nurse program, but at Inova systematically undermined it, visited me to discuss creating a nurse advice line because Inova's managed care contracts and affiliated physicians wanted a nursing triage service. I refused to work with him. Before joining Inova, he had specialized in selling potato chips for an advertising agency in Texas. He had had no experience in health care administration, let alone any clinical experience. He was fired not long afterward, but he never should have been hired.

When Inter+Net began to look hapless, I transferred most of my time to the Department of Health Services Research at Inova Health System that had been established to employ me. We had two large successes in the grand scheme of things, plus many smaller frustrations. The two successes occurred after I identified projects that I could control by myself, without outside interference by other department directors. About 1990, Inova Health System leaders said they wanted Inova to become an "integrated delivery system." I thought I knew what that was— something like Kaiser-Permanente, with physicians, facilities, and financial services all integrated to manage clinical and financial needs for health care services for defined populations of people over time. Because I believed that most of the hospital administrators and physicians in northern Virginia knew nothing about integrated care, I suggested that Inova sponsor a national meeting on the Future of

Integrated Health Care Systems to bring others from around the nation to teach us what integrated health care services really meant. Knox Singleton liked the idea. We partnered with The Healthcare Forum to cosponsor the meeting and to help us with program development and logistics. The idea led to four years of this conference, and we taught hundreds of key managers and physicians in Inova Health System what we meant by integrated health care without lecturing to them ourselves.

The other success was harder to achieve but potentially far more valuable to Inova. I learned about relational databases in the late 1980s. The technologies for storing data in a relational database management system were developed in research laboratories at IBM in the late 1970s and were introduced into a commercial product of IBM called DB/2 in the early 1980s. Quickly, competing systems appeared, from start-up companies with names such as Oracle, Sybase, Informix, and others. Oracle is now the second largest software vendor in the world, after Microsoft. Microsoft sells the leading relational database management system for personal computers, Access. Worldwide, hundreds of billions of dollars of license fees and payroll costs are devoted each year to information systems based on relational database management systems. I thought the technology might help Inova.

About 1991, I reasoned that computers were becoming much more powerful and less expensive, and relational technologies more robust. I argued that Inova should invest in a relational data warehouse devoted to storing a copy in electronic form of every piece of information about every patient ever seen in electronic form in any transaction system used within the Inova system, so we could study those data at our convenience, looking systematically for opportunities for quality improvement. It made sense that the Department of Health Services Research and Development would ask for such a resource. Information Systems employed no one at the time who knew anything about relational databases, and they were already up to their ears in requests for interfaces to existing transaction systems. The director of IS said he did not have the budget and did not have the staff to spare (the existing staff would not have known what to do anyway). He was not interested in "Marshall's toy." The Department of Information Systems was in the business of operating batch processing computer systems. They had very little to do with information services. Their job descriptions, which defined their universe of interests, did not include helping managers and physician executives obtain data for quality improvement. In fact, Marketing ran the cost accounting system. Information Systems was not involved in decision support systems. Most of the administrators and IS staff had never performed research of any kind, let alone retrospective observational data analysis.

Not to be overcome by the torpor and rigor of IS, I enlisted the support of leading physicians by promising them that we could eliminate most of the time wasted dredging clinical data from paper records. Administrators do not see the time physicians spend in Medical Records, either completing charts or rummaging through medical records for quality assurance reviews, as a cost to their institutions, so they are quite content to allow "the system" to squander physicians' time. Nurses' time is a cost to their institutions. So they do not want nurses abstracting charts unless necessary to keep the JCAHO content. But physicians' time, who cares?

I alerted the chiefs of medicine, surgery, psychiatry, cardiovascular surgery, and trauma that the pharmaceutical and laboratory data they were accustomed to exhuming from paper records were in fact briefly in electronic form in their transaction systems, usually long enough to copy them to another database for integration with other data on the same patients and then to permanent electronic storage. The clinical chiefs liked the idea of an electronic database for retrospective analysis and urged administration to fund a pilot test of the concept. We built a relational data warehouse in Sybase, using a natural language processor (Knowledge Base Management System) for the client interface. We incorporated data from the hierarchical cardiovascular surgery database written in MUMPS, as well as cost information from the cost accounting system and accounting details for the same patients.

We showed the system in more than a dozen meetings of physicians and administrators and conveyed to them that the technology for easy-to-use analytical systems based on relational data warehouses with client-server architecture was mature. We received the support of the organization to continue to develop the system, with a five-year budget of $7 million. We started the development project with Andersen Consulting but planned to include Inova staff on the project as soon as possible.

With funding approved by senior management and the board of Inova Health System, we moved the Department of Health Services Research and Development (HSR&D) to a new building, where we had about 4,000 square feet of space for about 25 people at our peak, most from Andersen Consulting. We worked tirelessly on the IRIS (Inova Research Information System) project. In Inova's Department of HSR&D we had a PhD psychologist, a nurse with systems development experience, a statistician, and clerical help. We tried to help managers and physicians analyze data. We concentrated on building the data warehouse and the annual national conference entitled "The Future of Integrated Health Care Systems."

As the leader of HSR&D, I made many mistakes. We did not lead Information Systems to support the data warehouse project in the first place and alienated them for several years by hiring Anderson Consulting. We did not go out into the operating units—hospitals and clinics—to show managers and physicians how to collect and analyze data. We remained too insular, focused on the grand decision support system. And the organization waited and waited.

We realized our mistake in alienating Information Systems when we needed their cooperation to write interfaces to the IRIS database. We realized the mistake of not proactively teaching the organization to collect and analyze data when our largest potential customer, Fairfax Hospital, created a department of Quality Improvement and Outcomes Studies, as if to say HSR&D does no good or is not available. We concentrated on bigger things and neglected the much larger importance of the vast number of small projects we could have been doing for clinicians and managers of Inova. We did not go to them or create a curriculum that would teach them the value of Health Services Research and Development.

After we had spent nearly $1,000,000 working on the client interface to IRIS, using Knowledge Base Management System (KBMS), I knew that it would not suffice to allow managers and physicians to pose any but the simplest queries to the system by themselves. I worried that the client inferface to such a complex database would make or break the system, since it was designed to give clinicians and managers direct access to a vast amount of patient-specific, detailed clinical and financial data for decision support. At the same time, in 1993, the income to Inova facilities was not growing as fast as operating expenses. One hospital had just closed after losing an important contract with a major insurer in greater Washington, and hundreds of middle managers found themselves looking for jobs outside of Inova. In that climate, I assumed I would not receive any more money than budgeted for the IRIS project.

Then Microsoft released Microsoft Access, named for its purpose, to serve as the client software for personal computers that give users access to their corporate data. It was designed to connect to corporate relational databases via ODBC (Open Database Connectivity standards) and allow users at their PCs to run queries on corporate data warehouses and extract data from them to their PCs for further analysis. In Access I saw an ideal client interface to the IRIS database, and I decided that we would have to abandon the interface work with KBMS and switch to Access, with substantial attendant incremental costs in the short term. This was near the first of the year, 1993, and I had to have a working system ready for inspection by June 1993 if I hoped to continue receiving funding for the project.

At this point I made another managerial mistake. I decided that, if I asked to spend more money than budgeted in the remainder of the fiscal year (six months) in order to substitute Access for KBMS, the manager to whom I then reported (the Chief Operating Officer of Inova) would not appreciate my motives and would tell me to live within my budget. On the other hand, I knew that I could not have a working system with Access as the front end with the funds then remaining in my budget. So I decided that I would spend one year's budget in those next six months, and create a system with Access at the front end that would wow the audience. Then I would ask forgiveness, since I believed they would like what they saw, and persuade them that I had saved money in the long run by reducing training costs for the system by substituting Access for KBMS.

Anyone who has survived to reach the top of a bureaucracy knows you do not surprise your boss as I did. When the evaluation came, everyone liked the Access client software more than KBMS, they believed that I had probably reduced the total cost of the system by substituting Access, and they even accepted my argument that I had simply spent money allocated for next year in this year to improve the overall product. I do believe that I would not have been allowed to spend the money to integrate Access into IRIS in the time I had to make the system functional before the review. I probably did save the project. But at a price to me.

I was not fired, but, behind the scenes, my budgetary authority was stripped and I became a titular head of the department, with the budget placed in the hands of the nurse who had reported to me. Her reporting relationship was changed to report to the CIO, as was mine. She and I became administrative peers. I had not had faith in my boss, and he had lost faith in my administrative judgment.

My interests turned outside of Inova. I had succeeded in proving the concept of a data warehouse and had ensured its continued development. I did not want to make a career at Inova. By summer 1993, I knew that I needed to find another purpose. I had four sons to educate. I knew I had to take a risk and build a business that might grow into a livelihood more financially rewarding than remaining an employee of a large health care bureaucracy. I turned my attention to ways I could become independent of Inova and of any other job such as I had at Inova. I did not want to make a lateral move to another health care organization, to battle with administrators in another setting. I wanted to start a business and change the face of health care services for the country. Entrepreneurial challenges and rewards appealed to me. I thought I could contribute much more to society than I had been able to produce at Inova. What could I do? I sensed an answer from my work for the American College of Physician Executives.

The American College of Physician Executives

Each of us needs a professional home where we can mingle with others like us in training and in goals. Most professionals rely on one, or more, professional associations for a sense of community of like-minded individuals from whom we can learn about the trials and tribulations, rewards and successes of pursuing our professions. ACPE became my haven. ACPE, now among the fastest growing professional associations in the house of medicine, in 1997 included some 13,000 physicians involved in the management of health care organizations. Most members of the ACPE hold the rank of medical director, vice president of medical affairs, managing partner, or chief executive officer. Most members join the ACPE in mid-career, in their 40s or 50s, after considerable clinical practice, to learn management techniques they can apply to their work as leaders. With an MBA and an MPH before I joined the ACPE, I was one of the youngest members, with more formal education in management than most members. I enjoyed the camaraderie of physicians who could share stories about obdurate boards, risk-averse administrators, and impulsive physicians. In so many basic ways, every hospital is like every other in the personalities of its administrators, board members, and physicians, and the stereotypes carry more than a seed of truth.

My interest in informatics led me to create a brief course of four hours on the subject for members of the ACPE. I taught the course in 1991 to a warm reception. The College had a model then of half-day courses and two-day courses, and not much in between. During the preparation for a two-day course entitled Introduction to Informatics to be presented in the summer of 1993, I realized I had enough material related to databases to add a second two-day course with hands-on exercises in database manipulation. ACPE took a gamble that the four days of classes would sell, and we offered them first in August 1993 in Boston to sold-out audiences. Since then, we have taught these programs three times per year and always have sold out our capacity. ACPE made the Introduction to Informatics a requirement for physicians to become certified in medical management.

By the middle of 1994, the Executive Vice President of ACPE, Roger Schenke, and I heard from members of the ACPE that they would like to introduce their senior executives to these two courses, but, because the courses fill with college members, they could not do so. We discussed creating an independent institute for informatics to teach courses in applied informatics to all members of the health care community. I presented to the board of directors of the ACPE a business plan for such an institute, and the board agreed to help promote what we called The Informatics Institute to members. I incorporated two companies in the State of Virginia in the summer of 1994, The Informatics Institute as a not-for-profit company and Ruffin Informatics, Inc., as a for-profit company that would manage The Informatics Institute.

We decided to market The Informatics Institute with a subscription to courses offered in the future, selling subscriptions to five courses for $2,750. The business plan included financial scenarios for subscribing 100, 200, 300, and 400 organizations. Of course, my optimism lead me to expect more than 400 organizations would subscribe, but my training at Stanford told me to plan for the worst. We decided that we could not make a go of The Informatics Institute with fewer than 200 subscribing organizations and still pay rent and salaries. With high hopes, ACPE promoted The Informatics Institute to its members in summer 1994. Unfortunately, due to delays all along the way in creation of the brochure, we mailed it during July while many people were on vacation and after most organizations had established their budgets for education for the following year.

By late August, we had obtained only about 75 subscriptions. I had reasonable assurances from Inova Health System that we could use part of the space in the Department of Informatics for our staff (of two to start) if we could not afford to rent space. Still imbued with optimism, I had selected attractive space in a modern office building adjacent to a new Ritz Carlton hotel but could not obtain a lease because the lessor wanted the lease cosigned by ACPE. Understandably, the ACPE would not cosign the lease. We set a date of September 15, 1994, for a go/no go decision on The Informatics Institute. If Inova permitted me and my secretary to stay in Inova space and start The Informatics Institute using Inova educational facilities, we would start the project with me and my secretary the only full-time employees as long as we had 100 subscribing organizations, giving us a nest egg of $275,000. On a rainy, cold September 20, 1994, I met with the Executive Vice President of ACPE, Roger Schenke, at a Washington, D.C., hotel where the ACPE had a meeting. He told me later he expected me to back out of the project, and ACPE would refund the subscriptions to members. That day we had 101 subscribing organizations.

I wanted to create The Informatics Institute and Ruffin Informatics. I could estimate the expense of educating my four sons through graduate school, and I wanted to offer them the kind of education my father had provided me. Entrepreneurship is in me. I knew I could not afford such an education on the salary I earned as a clinical information officer or a medical director. Working in a bureaucracy and attending countless meetings where staff jockeyed for position and prestige at the expense of the organization depressed me. So, I said to Roger that I would create The Informatics Institute, but the ACPE needed to give me time to pay back the value of the promotion it had invested in The Informatics Institute. I would make The Informatics Institute for-profit, with me as the owner. I would not take such a risk with my career without the opportunity for ownership. I took a cut in pay and established Ruffin Informatics, Inc., to do business as The Informatics Institute.

We discussed these arrangements with the board of the ACPE. They saw the benefit to the profession of medical management of The Informatics Institute but also saw the risk to me personally. They wished me well. Inova Health System gave me space in which we could work and teach in return for a substantial discount on the price Inova paid for courses, and we started the business..

The Informatics Institute

By the end of our first year of operations, we had sold about 170 subscription, far fewer than we had hoped. We had added one other staff person, a systems analyst from Inova with experience in respiratory therapy, to help me with course development, but we did not have the resources to market The Informatics Institute. We were stuck with insufficient capital to market our services or move to our own office space. The ACPE created and mailed promotional literature in fall 1995, but it produced many fewer subscriptions than the advertising of one year earlier had produced. Instead of the first subscriptions being the tip of a much larger iceberg, as I had hoped, I faced the daunting prospect that we had instead picked all the low-hanging fruit with the first advertising and that getting more subscribers would cost much more money, which we did not have. By winter, 1996, things looked grim. I had recruited two employees from Inova by giving them substantial raises. We were spending more money than we were taking in subscriptions. We did not have the cash to advertise.

About this time, I talked about my hopes for The Informatics Institute with a life-long friend, John Redmond. We were in school together through high school, then went our separate ways. We saw each other infrequently while John attended college in New Hampshire and business school at the University of Chicago and worked on Wall Street in futures trading and banking. John's love is starting businesses, which I learned at our 20th high school reunion in 1990. I told him then of my interest in computers in medicine and my wish to start a company. He had moved back to Washington and was in the process of starting a biotechnology company.

We kept in touch after the reunion, and, in fall 1995, we began to talk in earnest about opportunities for The Informatics Institute. He knew we were undercapitalized and could tell I did not know how to run a small business. He sold a business he was operating at the time and agreed to consult for me. Quickly he saw that my two employees and I had little experience with the trials and tribulations of a start-up. We spent money as if we were still employed by Inova. Because cash was getting very low, John offered to join the company as employee and owner, and invested needed cash to keep us going. Quickly John implemented business processes that we had not had, including accounting and payroll systems. He brought in an accountant part time to keep our books accurately.

By June 1996, The Informatics Institute had sold nearly 200 subscriptions, but cash was very tight. We worried we could not afford office space, but we knew we had to sever the umbilical cord to Inova and find our own office space. We created 10 two-day courses, using consultants I knew to be competent teachers for four of the courses and physician executives for six courses, including four that I taught. The physicians invested more time and effort in the teaching materials than the consultants were willing to invest. The consultants kept audiences interested with their anecdotes but would not produce the detailed, annotated materials that I wanted to become a hallmark of The Informatics Institute. I knew that the Institute had to graduate from its dependence on outside consultants for faculty, but the consultants wanted to get in front of the audience and did not require honoraria.

In summer 1996, several large health care organizations requested that The Informatics Institute teach its courses on site so they could send more people to attend the courses than they could fly to our facility. John and I saw an opportunity for growth without substantial marketing expenses. We contracted to teach for UniHealth in Los Angeles, Catholic Healthcare West in San Francisco, and Methodist Hospital in Indianapolis, and Inova continued to contract with us to teach its managers and affiliated physicians. With these corporate contracts, we earned a more predictable revenue stream and could schedule courses that others could take as well in those cities. Unfortunately, we did not have the funds to advertise our programs in those cities, except from our Web site. Nevertheless, we did have some students from other parts of the United States and Canada attend our courses in Los Angeles, San Francisco, Indianapolis, and Washington.

By fall 1996, we had enough business to give us some confidence we could move into our own space for teaching and offices. We considered the entire metropolitan Washington area and finally decided on modest accommodations in a great location. We wanted to appeal to local students and students who might fly in from out of town. We selected space in Bethesda, Maryland, adjacent to the National Library of Medicine and the National Institutes of Health, across the street from three hotels and a subway stop, in Bethesda's restaurant district. Our location gives students three airports to use, including Baltimore—Washington International. Making that move signaled the maturation of our company to an infant stage, out of the incubator that Inova's office and training space gave us. We have to watch cash flow carefully and gauge carefully when we can expect cash payments from our corporate clients.

By fall 1997, we were adding organizations with which we contract, teaching in more venues, planning conferences and a data warehouse for students, and hoping to add more staff, including another physician to support course development and teaching. We know what we want to do. We want to become a knowledge business disseminating expertise by course work, distance learning, and self-paced computer tutorials to help the health care industry learn how to use digital information processing and communication technologies to take care of patients and to operate their organizations more efficiently and effectively. What I learned in business school certainly is apt today. Execution is everything.

Chapter 11

Insurance Company Medical Director

by Ruth Pagano, MD, MBA, FACPE

The following tribute was recently delivered by one of my Fallon Clinic partners during an award ceremony at St. Vincent's Hospital to mark my 25 years of clinical service:

"When Ruth Pagano was selected as Senior Medical Director of Blue Cross Blue Shield of Connecticut last year, she became only the third woman in the nationwide Blue Cross Association to hold such a position. When she was installed April 1996 as a Fellow in the American College of Physician Executives joining an elite group of 312 men and six other women, it also was not the first time she was a pioneer. When she left her Chicago home in 1963 to start medical school at St. Louis University, Ruth Ann Fazioli, the oldest of 7 children, joined three other female classmates and 120 men in pursuing the intense studies that would begin her clinical career in pediatrics.

"She came East when she matched as an intern for the Children's Service at the Massachusetts General Hospital with a salary of $1,000 a year, the reward for the privilege of working long hours and every other night on call for two straight years. During her residency at Boston Children's hospital , she met Matteo Pagano, a teacher and principal in the Shrewsbury, Massachusetts, school system. That started their 27-year marriage partnership that would bring her to Worcester and to motherhood of two sons, Matthew and Thomas. One is a lawyer in Chicago, the other a PhD graduate student in Arizona. Staying in Boston during their first year of marriage, Ruth became a fellow at Harvard in Primary Care Medicine, working in a community health clinic in Roxbury and teaching medical students, including the now famous Michael Critchton of "ER" fame.

"In 1971, she joined a new multispecialty group practice, another pioneering move, to become its 14th member and 2nd women. Along with her partners, Drs. John Duggan and John Riordan, Ruth built the pediatric practice and eventual Fallon Pediatric Department into the complex and very popular place for care in Worcester that it still is today. She was chosen to initiate new practices in many of Fallon's satellites dotting Central Massachusetts. Leadership roles, such as Chairman of the utilization review committee, Chief of Pediatrics, and member of the Board of Directors of Fallon Community Health Plan, gave her a taste for administration. She generously donated her time managing the medical care of foreign children brought to Worcester through the Heal the Children and CHANGE organizations. She loved studying international health systems, having been to China, Italy, and Latin America.

"In 1989, while spending nights at Clark University in a Masters Program, Ruth was chosen as a Kron Scholar, enabling her to go to North Carolina to study medical management at the Kenan Business School. It was there, under the tutelage of mentors such as Drs. John Meyers, Joel Kauffman, and Bob Cavanaugh, that she decided that she wanted to be a medical director. She passed the examination for the American Board of Medical Management and finished her MBA in Health Care Administration, knowing she would need these credentials in this challenging field.

"Moving was a very difficult decision for Ruth and her family to make when she was offered the opportunity to become the North East Regional Medical Director for Travelers Insurance Company in Hartford in spring 1994, as she would have to leave the Fallon Clinic after 24 years of service. She really missed her patients and colleagues. But the next two years brought new learning about the insurance business and benefits administration and the opportunity of working with some excellent nurse managers.

"After the merger of Travelers and MetLife Health networks, she moved on to Blue Cross, settling into a new medical directorship as Director of the Utilization and Case Management Department in North Haven, Connecticut, responsible for more than a half million covered lives. Her managerial roles have been made easier by using many of the managed care principles she learned from expert health care administrators such as Christy Bell and Alan Stoll. We wish her as much success in her second career as health care administrator as she achieved in her first clinical career."

The next day I received a call to contribute this chapter about the value of the MBA to one's career as a physician executive. This testimonial sets the background against which my second career was possible because of the MBA experience.

The Need for Management Training
Kron Management Scholarship

Dr. Alan Kronhaus, CEO of Kron Physicians, a locum tenens company, recognized the increasing need for business training for physicians, whether they were just finishing a residency, managing an active clinical practice, or playing a major administrative role in their current organizations. In 1989, he approached the Kenan Business School at the University of North Carolina at Chapel Hill and proposed an executive training program for physicians interested in management. These week-long seminar-style classes would be supplemented with team projects, the case study method, evening lectures by medical care administrators, and independent study spread over eight months. This six-session course would give an opportunity for student physicians to prepare homework between monthly course work, apply business principles learned in class to their current situation, and do an organizational survey on their present work environments. Each student would have an advisor to develop a business plan project.

Dr. Kronhaus facilitated tuition reimbursement opportunities by offering clinical and administrative locum tenens monthly internships for these physicians to investigate new areas of professional interest in different institutions. After screening a hundred applicants to the program, he welcomed his first Kron Scholars to Chapel Hill in August 1990. Twenty-two physicians from diverse backgrounds, representing the medical novice and the experienced practitioner, gathered from every region in the United States for a unique adventure. Hand-picked Kenan Business School professors provided the didactic work. Joanne Cretella, the academic dean, organized not only academic but also social programs and evening guest speakers. Alan, an entrepreneur extraordinaire, motivated the group into exploring all the aspects of managerial skills necessary for physician executives. He catalyzed the group into work teams that looked forward to their reunion very 5 weeks. Later, he formalized this program as the current CompHealth Physician Executive training program.

Being a member of that premier Kron Scholar class led me to the most rewarding exploratory opportunity of my career. To hear the experiences of solo practitioners from New Jersey and Arkansas and to study with a vice president medical affairs in Cleveland, a Californian HMO staff physician, and a physician just named president of a PHO enriched the experience. We listened to lawyers and politicians who were legislating the Medical Practitioner Data Bank Act and to public health officials struggling with health care reform. Yes, it was hard sacrificing all my annual vacation time to fly every fifth week to North Carolina in addition to finding coverage for my busy adolescent practice. I remember one Mother' s Day when I needed to turn down a dinner invitation from my sons to finish up a paper due that week.

In June 1991, I took a modified "leave of absence" from my Fallon practice to go to LaPorte Hospital in Indiana to shadow Lee Morris, the hospital administrator. I earned my Kron tuition by taking pediatric night call that month. Next, I worked a month at Harvard Community Health Plan in Boston as assistant medical director, learning the CO-STAR computerized medical record, how a staff-model HMO functioned, how the plan paid its physicians, and what performance standards they required. Several hours a day, I substituted for the Chief of Pediatrics, who was on his honeymoon in Europe. Returning from those two experiences gave me the incentive to drive headlong into finishing my MBA classes, filling in my gaps in knowledge. I now knew my goal was to be a physician executive.

The Role of ACPE

Members and the staff of the American College of Physician Executives (formerly the American College of Medical Directors) played a vital role in my career transition from a clinician to a health care administrator. I remember a Career Transition workshop with George and Barbara Linney where an OB-Gyn specialist suggested to me that hospital administration is very hierarchy-dependent and that usually surgical and medical specialists move up that ladder much faster than pediatricians. Being a female pediatrician also probably put me on the bottom wrung. Perhaps I should consider a goal other than CEO of a hospital in my future. Why not leverage my experience in managed care and my board work in the health insurance industry and consider being a insurance medical director? The Women's Forum, a small group of physician executive "wannabes" who meet at ACPE meetings, enabled me to network with other women already in executive and administrative positions, such as Drs. Deborah Hammond, Randy Ellis, Toni Mitchell, and Deborah Shlian (see chapter 12). These sessions were a guiding inspiration for which I am thankful. Wes Curry, editor of *Physician Executive* was very helpful to me as I wrote on managed care topics.

The Importance Of Mentoring

In 1990, I was matched with Dr. Alfredo Czerwinski, Medical Director of the Kelsey Seybold Clinic, in a year-long American College of Physician Executives Mentoring Program. We had been chosen as a preceptor-observer pair because of the similar sizes of our multispecialty group practices. After my field trip to Houston and his return visit to Worcester, the year passed very quickly. His mentoring began to have serious implications for my future choices. We held monthly teleconferences and exchanged frequent letters on important happenings in our mutual organizations. He gave me managerial assignments and made me reflect on what skills I would need that he, as a medical director possessed. It was easy to see what makes him so successful. He is a great teacher and coach.

Crisis Point

Would it be conceivable that a pioneer member of the Fallon Clinic group practice might consider leaving after 24 years, with all the success and positive reputation of that organization, and start a new career? Why would one want to leave a comfortable practice with plenty of partners. Shouldn't this be the time for golfing or pleasures with one's family? Only another easy 10 years would lead to a lucrative retirement. Why would one risk the insurance industry, especially when Hillary Clinton's reform bill had just been proposed.

The Value of an MBA in the Health Insurance Industry

Some define managed care as the application of business principles to the health care industry. What better preparation can one have than a concentrated study of business administration to bring that training to the managed care marketplace. After 24 years of successful pediatric and adolescent medical practice, it seemed a strange decision to return to the classroom. The strongest imperative necessitating this direction was my simultaneous appointment as Chief of Pediatrics and a member of the Board of Directors of the HMO insurance health plan associated with our group practice. I had always been interested in management issues, preparing the on-call schedule for 35 of us, holding team meetings with the nursing staff, reading the details of the annual reports of the hospital, and monitoring patient accounts receivables. But giving feedback to departmental physicians about their individual productivity and behavior, making salary recommendations to the treasurer based on physicians' performance, negotiating the political interplay between the employees of the practice and the administrators, and having to facilitate others' job satisfaction sent me right smack into the world of personnel management and organizational behavior. Luckily, my first MBA course was in organizational behavior.

The Educational Decision

Living in a community with a medical school has many advantages—not only the best of grand rounds, but also the opportunity to stay abreast of current advances in one's field and to teach medical students and residents. There was also the proximity of the Harvard School of Public Health. I had always been interested in the "bigger picture," and being a member of the community faculty gave me the opportunity to take graduate courses free. These included biostatistics, community health education, epidemiology, how to write a scientific article, and health care economics. Here I was enjoying teaching future doctors and satisfying my own thirst for "continuous learning."

One semester, Don Berwick, MD, and the TQM bug bit the University of Massachusetts Academic Medical Center. Students from a neighboring university's health care administration program flooded into my public health course on CQI projects in the hospital setting. Being on several project teams with them, I came to know a group of students who were striving to make a difference in the future of health care delivery. That is when I decided to enroll in the university's master's program, just to be able to continue to relate to these future administrators.

It was the early 1990s and computerization was just taking serious hold in the health care world. Computerization of medical records, patient accounts, and practice management systems was bringing vendors right into the office in the middle of clinical time. In addition, I was learning their language at medical management conventions. Thank goodness my next class was on management information systems. My sons and the Worcester Mac Users group also introduced me to the competency I have today with mainframes, PCs, my handy laptop spreadsheets, medical informatics, and the world of the Internet.

My financial accounting class taught me a lot more than how to read a balance sheet and the *Wall Street Journal* or to figure a break-even point. It also helped me to understand the headaches of our treasurer and accountants. I learned how to do cost-benefit analyses, calculate return on investment, know the difference between fixed and variable costs, and understand profit margin. Preparing my $5 million department budget this year was also made easier because of this course. Marketing classes were full of case studies in other industries, but what I learned about competitive force analysis, advertising, image making techniques, and customer market segmentation have been some of the most needed competencies as the health care insurance industry soon learned that brokers are our distribution channels and how to be nice to them.

A quality assurance course was most instructive about quality of medical care in hospitals and taught me the lesson of doing things right the first time. My next class—TQM principles, CQI projects, and tools—opened for me the whole world of customer service and client satisfaction that has became the underpinnings of the National Committee for Quality Assurance (NCQA) accreditation process. We studied the criteria of the Malcolm Baldrige Awards. Since then, I have participated in NCQA accreditation visits for two organizations that have achieved full three-year accreditation status. Group activities and exercises in teamwork were essential as I transitioned from a fiercely independent practitioner to a team player with a cross-functional staff.

Meanwhile integrated health care systems that were emerging from synergistic mergers in our medical community gave me practical material to write research papers in a course on mergers and acquisitions. Consolidation of local hospitals that rarely communicated with each other became an everyday news event. Our market share and success as a group model HMO appeared to have peaked, and decisions about partnerships and alliances became a practical necessity. That class helped me to better understand the transition steps and the need for "change agents" as we work through the merger mania characteristic of the health care insurance industry today.

My class on legal aspects of health care administration rewarded me with all of the latest information on malpractice, vicarious liability, "any willing provider" laws, resistance, and advanced directives. I came to know the need for due diligence. Because I had served for years on an active board of directors, budget preparation, benefit management, risk management, strategic planning, and quality assurance came as second nature to me. These committees gave me practical experience and the opportunity to make each class come alive as I applied the principles I learned at night to the day-to-day operations of our organization. All those classes on strategy and tactical planning and project management paid off in interpreting the piles of task plans and Gantt charts on my desk today. Breakthrough thinking, stakeholders, key success factors, and balanced scorecards became my new vocabulary.

Negotiation and contracting was one of my most valuable courses. Needing to negotiate professional and institutional contracts, fee schedules and risk-sharing arrangements, as well as to assure myself the best salary possible, was well worth the practice sessions. Learning to sit and listen and observe body language was a struggle for this strong-willed physician. Learning to prioritize and to delegate were lessons number two and three.

One of my final MBA classes was entitled "Human Resource Management, Diversity in the Workplace and Affirmative Action." It was a challenging but very revealing class. I came to realize that health care has a very female-dominated workforce, until you get into administration. Writing the affirmative action plan for the Fallon Clinic was an interesting exercise and gave me new insight into exploring the barriers to promotion and the power struggles in health care field. I came to know that becoming a medical director, less than 10 percent of whom are women, would not be easy. All this is happening at a time when understanding cultural diversity is vital to promotion of healthy life-styles and ideal medical care.

Preparing a résumé, practicing interviewing techniques, writing performance appraisals, creating transition plans for employees during a merger, working with an outplacement organization, and establishing mock severance packages would later be needed as I supervised increasingly larger groups of employees over the next three to four years. Little would I realize the personal impact of mergers and downsizing until one year into my new job. Graduation day finally arrived on May 15, 1994, and, with it, the reward of a contract for a new position signed two weeks before the ceremony.

Insurance Medical Director

What is it like to be an insurance medical director? The image of the retired doctor pushing papers from behind a desk, making unilateral decisions, and searching claims for fraud is fading fast. Nearly every health care insurance company today, managed care or not, relies heavily on one or more medical directors who are directly communicating with providers and insurance administrators on a daily basis. Many of them are managing large utilization review and quality assurance nursing staff, performing direct catastrophic case management, establishing disease management programs, acting as members of sales teams at Fortune 500 companies, and facing political and legislative concerns. Most are on risk management panels as well as credentialing committees.

Some days are long and frustrating. Taking frequent calls from providers whose services are interpreted as not being medically necessary can be a challenge. One must comb the research literature and the latest technological assessments to determine whether a new procedure or drug would make this request experimental or investigational. One shares medical expertise when appeals are made against unpaid claims. One may need to administer a medical policy or benefit decision that may not be that customer friendly, to patient or doctor. One may need to talk to the media about a company's experience with "drive through" mastectomies and risk being misquoted in the process.

Rewards

But there are rewards. Such as reviewing a complex clinical situation with the case manager who just coordinated the care of a patient with congestive heart failure, avoiding another hospitalization by sending out the "IV Lasix nurse" just in time. Or being able to sign off on hundreds of clean credentialing packages of a network that meets the geographical access needs of the marketing department. It is nice attending a contracting meeting with a hospital CFO who characterizes your team as really "tough." Other days are fulfilling, such as when the HEDIS data rolls in with marked improvement over last year's figures and you can send out some excellent provider report cards. You will long remember the day you heard cheering outside your door when word came of the full three-year NCQA accreditation. There is also plenty of opportunity to travel to local and national meetings to benchmark with colleagues whom you now number in the administrative as well as the clinical ranks.

New Competencies

Did a medical degree and several years of clinical experience give me the credentials to understand the health insurance industry, or did an MBA teach me the mechanism of insurance and the principles of managed care? I remember the remarks of Dan Cave, Vice President of Product Development and Marketing, who hired me into my first full-time medical directorship. "You should know I am buying your MBA, since now we can speak the same language." His words return to me every once in a while when I get teased about no longer being a "real doctor" or about having gone over to the "other side" as an insurance company medical director.

The motto at Anthem Blue Cross and Blue Shield of Connecticut—"Our Plan Is to Keep You Healthy"—reflects our stated mission to provide the best value for the health care dollar. By identifying consumer wants and requirements, we are able to set competitive rates and manage benefit products, pricing, and operations so as to continuously improve member care and the health of the population we serve. I am certainly proud to be a member of this organization today.

As an insurance company medical director, I believe that my influence on health care is much broader than it was in clinical practice. Personal rewards also come from the foundation changes realized through the MBA experience. Several years have passed since my transition to medical administration. As I reflect on the journey, certainly the MBA educational experience was supplemented by contact with other professionals making similar life changes. Advisors, mentors, and coaches may be available for others in their own organizations, but, for me, the process of obtaining that diploma made all the difference in my career.

Chapter 12

Management Search Firm President and CEO

by Deborah Shlian, MD, MBA

"Two roads diverged in a wood, and I—I took the one less traveled by, And that has made all the difference.—Robert Frost, The Road Not Taken.

I was fortunate enough to hear Robert Frost himself speak those words when my mother took me to a literary seminar at Johns Hopkins University. Although it was long ago (I was in grade school), I remember very clearly the message I took from that brilliant poet: it was okay to be different, to explore possibilities and options others might not, to "do your own thing." Growing up in the late 1950s and early 1960s, a time when family and career roles were still fairly rigidly differentiated by gender, this view required adjustments from parents, friends, and particularly school counselors, who regarded nursing or teaching as much more acceptable careers for women than medicine. Indeed, the idea of career itself was "something to fall back on," to be dusted off should a husband die or family economics really get tight. Full-time wife and mother was the generally accepted proper role for a woman of that era. Needless to say, I took Frost's words to heart, starting with aiming for a medical career early in life and then by taking various forks in the path as opportunities presented themselves. And that, for me, has made all the difference.

The First Fork

The first fork came at the end of medical school, when I had to make a decision about specializing. In 1972, although there had been some brief mention of family practice as a new specialty, there were very few residencies in the country and even less guidance as to where to find them—particularly on the East Coast. So, despite my fascination with the concept of a "new, complete physician," I chose the road of least resistance and matched with a Hopkins radiology training program. It was a chance vacation to Los Angeles during my internship year that changed the course of my clinical career. My husband (we married in my junior year of medical school) arranged for a meeting with the head of family medicine at Kaiser Permanente. Our preventive medicine curriculum in medical school had included a comprehensive study of what was considered by many traditionalists to be a renegade operation (or worse, socialized medicine), i.e., a group-model health maintenance organization. The notion of salaried doctors working in a prepaid multispecialty group that functioned as a partnership was different, if not heretical, in the 1970s, when the vast majority of doctors were in solo practice. But my husband and I had found the concept more than intellectually interesting. It seemed to make a lot of sense, and we were anxious to see the system up close.

Dr. Irv Rasgon was my first real role model and mentor. Chief of Family Medicine at the Sunset facility, he charmed us from the moment we met him. Irv was the quintessential Marcus Welby. He even looked the part. A great clinician, an outstanding teacher, and a natural leader, he was passionate about family practice and Kaiser. "Why specialize and become so narrowly focused when you can be a family practitioner and take care of the whole patient?" he asked us. Irv took us on hospital rounds, and his patients, from the very young to the very old, obviously adored him. Moreover, it was clear that his peers in other specialties respected him. When he offered us the opportunity to come to Los Angeles, finish our training as FPs and become Kaiser staff physicians, we readily accepted. I left radiology; my husband left ophthalmology; together we headed out to Southern California where we completed our training, took and passed family practice boards, and joined the Southern California Permanente Group as partners.

Looking back, the 10 years I spent as a clinician in the Kaiser group provided the kind of education in medicine and management that no didactic program in either medical or business school could ever provide. We were at the forefront of what has been nothing short of a revolution in health care, working in a fully integrated system that allowed us to deliver high-quality care (as much of the full spectrum of pediatric and adult medicine as was feasible in an urban hospital/clinic setting) without the stress of wondering whether our patients could pay for the care they required (what we know today as "managed care"). We had the advantage of being hospital-based, making our inpatients easily accessible during the day while we saw our scheduled outpatients in our offices, which were located in the same building. Similarly, we could often grab "sidewalk" consults from specialists who worked down the hall or just upstairs, thus avoiding long appointment delays for our patients. Laboratory, x-ray, and other ancillary services were a floor below—another efficiency. We were given a half day a week of "paid education time," which my husband and I used to teach residents at UCLA. Medical students from both UCLA and USC spent one-month electives at our Kaiser offices, and I was even able to satisfy my clinical research interests with such projects as a study of "Screening and Immunization of Rubella-Susceptible Women" that was published in *JAMA*.

My department held regular quality assurance and peer review sessions; we developed clinical guidelines long before they were fashionable. From a quality standpoint, I believed then and still believe today that the group model is an ideal way to practice medicine. Unfortunately, it is also extremely capital-intensive. In the highly competitive market that characterized California even in the 1980s, some of the original idealism began giving way to market pressures. As a primary care clinician, I became increasingly frustrated with my inability to influence policy. I felt that front-line physicians had the best perspective for identifying and correcting problems within the system. Yet, despite the fact that legally the group was a partnership, in reality it was governed no differently from most corporate entities, i.e., top down, and the top physician leaders were almost exclusively specialists. For example, the chief of my hospital was a surgeon who often stated that patients did not care about having their own physicians, that they were primarily motivated by easy access to the system, and that any clinician—doctor, nurse practitioner, or physician's assistant—would do just fine. It didn't matter. Needless to say, this undercut the fundamental principles of family medicine: taking care of the whole patient and being able to provide continuity of care by the same physician. In fact, this chief refused to accept the validity of our early studies (later, a group out of Vermont published the same findings) showing that patients with their own primary care doctors had fewer emergent visits and less inappropriate hospital admissions—both a significant cost savings and a quality improvement. Again, with hindsight, I now realize that his intransigence on this and other health care policy issues created an opportunity for me to take my next fork in the road; my husband and I both decided to leave Kaiser.

The Second Fork

With no one to provide career guidance, we began investigating how we could use our skills and understanding of health care to have a greater impact on the system. I wrote several articles, as well as a consumer health guide for a national health maintenance organization, and we both spoke at various venues around the country about problems involved with the delivery of care in the managed care environment. During the first few months of my "retirement," we were persuaded to start part-time law school at Whittier School of Law in Los Angeles, with the intention of developing an expertise in health policy and health law. However, not long after starting my first semester, I was recruited to a management position at the UCLA Student Health Service (SHS).

I became Director of the Primary Care Unit of SHS, which serves all 33,000 undergraduate and graduate students on the university campus. As many as 400 patients per day were being seen in our clinic, most of whom used Student Health as their only source of medical care. What attracted me to the position was the opportunity to take many of the lessons learned from the Kaiser system and adapt them to this setting. In particular, I wanted to change the orientation of primary care from essentially a triage area to a comprehensive ambulatory care facility staffed by clinicians competent enough to have admitting privileges at UCLA Medical Center. That meant letting nonboard-certified physicians go and hiring only well-credentialed family practitioners, pediatricians, and internists—a process fraught with legal/risk management personnel issues that I had to quickly research and understand. In addition, I wanted to integrate our service with the outstanding teaching programs in the medical school. That required developing a new level of diplomatic skill, delicately balancing the egos and agendas of various departments within the school. But happily, within a relatively short time, we had developed an impressive educational and research program that helped to attract medical students, graduate students, and superior clinical staff. Our quality of care and patient and personnel satisfaction all measurably improved.

As my administrative duties expanded, two significant issues surfaced that ultimately led to yet another fork in my career path. First was the question of whether I could be a successful manager and maintain a clinical practice without compromising both efforts. Increasingly, I felt caught between what I perceived as two equally important and demanding responsibilities. In the past, there seemed to be consensus that, despite the difficulties, one could not be an effective and credible leader of clinicians without concurrently having an active clinical practice. In fact, with the exception of a very few full-time regional medical directors, that is still the model Kaiser uses today for most of its physician administrators. On the other hand, in many other health care organizations, the role of physician executive has expanded so that those who wish to assume broad management responsibilities within these companies realize they must relinquish the clinical role, instead bringing the strong patient care background as a resource to a new, more comprehensive job description. Still, I must admit it was not an easy decision, although, looking back, it was one that has made all the difference in my success as a manager. As an executive who was also a physician, I was in the unique position of developing and enhancing collaboration and integration of the medical and administrative staffs in the daily management and operations of the organization.

The other issue had to do with my expanding operational responsibilities. Up to that point, everything I had accomplished as a manager was achieved without the benefit of a formal educational foundation. For example, I was asked to develop a budget, but I had never taken a finance or accounting course. I was asked to make staffing projections, but I had never learned the kind of operations research tools needed to create a truly robust model. Without a working knowledge of the language and concepts of business, one becomes totally reliant on nonmedical administrative personnel whose orientation to the bottom line may at least sometimes run counter to quality. This revelation convinced me to switch from law school to business school, and, in 1988, I completed an executive MBA program at UCLA's Anderson School of Management.

Two things occurred as a result of the MBA program. First, my job description expanded to include policy formulation, strategic planning, broader budgeting responsibilities, contracting for outside specialty care, risk management, and helping to develop and implement a computerized patient record to capture data for outcomes measurement. I became part of the senior management team, attending meetings heretofore open only to the nonphysician administrators.

Second, I began receiving telephone calls and letters from recruiters alerting me to other opportunities in medical management. Suddenly, I was advised that my experiences as both a clinician and manager in two managed care settings, coupled with my MBA degree, made me a strong candidate for many organizations looking to import that kind of expertise. Both flattered and curious, I decided to explore a few of these possibilities.

I had never worked with recruiters before and so had no idea what to expect. Someone would call my office, identify themselves as representing a particular job opportunity, and then inquire as to whether I wanted to be considered as a candidate. If not, did I know someone else who might. Surprisingly, the recruiter often had minimal information about the organization and asked few relevant questions about my management experience and none about my interests and career goals. Moreover, when I did interview, I often found the opportunity quite different from that described to me, from the nature of the job to the organization itself. It seemed clear that these recruiters were not serving their clients optimally. Sending inappropriate or disinterested candidates is a waste of time and money. However, as I have come to learn, even negative situations can become potential opportunities.

As a result of these disappointing searches, I suddenly realized that an unfilled niche existed: full-service, comprehensive search consulting in the managed care market. True, there were plenty of people out there calling themselves recruiters. But no other firm dealing in that specific market had someone with my credentials.

As a respected physician manager continually interfacing with the national medical community, I felt I could bring a unique perspective to searches. My credibility could further enhance a client company's reputation as I discussed available opportunities with prospective professional candidates. The other value-added component would be my willingness to develop long-term relationships with fellow physicians, guiding them through the search process, even putting some on the management career path initially and then mentoring them along the way. As I had personally experienced, no one in the search industry seemed interested in investing the kind of time (and thus capital) it takes to develop an executive's career, nor does anyone (as far as I know) have the kind of hands-on understanding of the talent pool to give appropriate advice.

The Third Fork

Despite the sense that I could do it better, it took many months of soul searching before I actually took the next fork in the road, eventually making the career transition from physician manager to medical management search consultant. My position at UCLA was tenured, I had spent six years developing staff and programs I believed in, I loved working with the students, and I had been told by my professors in the management school that more new businesses fail than succeed, especially consulting firms. According to a recent article in *Fortune* magazine, only one new consultancy in five will thrive.[1] If I really wanted to be an entrepreneur, I had to be willing to take that risk.

Armed with a business plan, including mission statement, I finally decided to take the plunge. Starting in 1990, I began to slowly build a firm that initially concentrated only on physician executive searches. As a career counselor to potential candidates, I often spent untold hours evaluating career goals and life priorities, reworking resumes, developing better interview techniques, and assisting with contract negotiations. The best payback has been the satisfaction of having launched many successful management careers, watching these individuals make significant contributions to a variety of health care organizations. Over time, my clients have requested broader services, so I have expanded my focus, becoming a consultant for established as well as start-up health plans, academic institutions, utilization review companies, research organizations, and even other health care consulting firms. I help these organizations build high-performance management teams by identifying appropriate entry-, middle- and senior- level nonphysician as well as physician management personnel vital for their success. That means fully understanding the organization, from governance to culture; evaluating specific personnel needs; conducting local and national salary surveys as the market changes; keeping close tabs on the interview process from start to finish, including contract negotiations; and following-up regularly with both the client company and new employee for at least a year after a placement is made to be sure an optimal transition has been achieved.

In 1994, my husband Joel joined me as President of the company. This year we incorporated as Shlian and Associates, Inc., moving our main base of operations to Florida while maintaining our West Coast office. Both Joel and I are active in professional health care organizations such as the American College of Physician Executives and the Group Health Association of America, always keeping abreast of changes in medicine and, in particular, managed care. We also regularly contribute articles and chapters for various textbooks on current management issues. Additionally, we have developed affiliations with more than a dozen associates with offices across the country, all with strong health care backgrounds, who we call upon to assist with specific searches. In this way, we are able to service our clients effectively while still maintaining the boutique nature of the company. Many small business owners feel compelled to expand in order to demonstrate success. However, according to Douglas Handler, an economist at Dun & Bradstreet, longevity rather than growth is the real measure of achievement. "Companies that last three years will usually make it," he claims. "Indeed, if you begin a company to capitalize on the wisdom and personal service of a key individual—namely you— big is bad. Adding staff and projects can spread the core value of your firm so thinly that customers are dissatisfied."[1] David Birch, founder of Cognetics, an economic analysis company noted for its studies of small firms says: "In the knowledge-based service firm, there are no economies of scale."[1]

After seven successful years, this seems to make sense. We continue to enjoy repeat business from clients who hire us knowing we are much more involved in the details, we personally know prospective candidates, and we can do the job more efficiently and less expensively than larger firms with high-rise offices and huge overheads. While a large firm may be able to coast on its reputation, Joel and I never can. If we perform poorly for clients, our business fails. Bottom line: being your own boss is definitely not for the faint of heart, but if your vision triumphs, the success is yours alone and therefore all the sweeter. For me, the shift from a management position in a highly bureaucratic and hierarchical organization to CEO of my own company has been the most exciting and positive experience of my professional life.

Conclusion

As a final word, I am constantly asked about the value of an MBA, particularly by physicians contemplating switching from clinical medicine to management. I can say with great confidence that for me, the MBA education and the degree itself have made all the difference in my career. As a manager, I was able to directly apply the classroom knowledge to my work, enabling me to expand my role to include much more of the business/operations side of the organization. As a search consultant, I regularly work directly with CEOs, CFOs, and COOs who appreciate the fact that I can speak their language. Often intimidated by physicians, they feel comfortable talking to a "fellow MBA." As the CEO of my own business, the training in accounting, finance, and marketing has been particularly useful.

Notwithstanding the value of a management education for me, I would advise any physician considering going back to school that an MBA will not provide the same kind of ticket that the MD did. By that I mean that having a business degree on your résumé, even from one of the elite schools, is not sufficient to land you a job as a manager, nor is it still generally required for most positions. What really counts is management experience and the ability to show that you have produced tangible results for an organization, often identified by such measures as greater market share, larger profits, decreased costs, reduced utilization, better outcomes, and increased patient satisfaction.

An MBA should never be viewed as the means to "get out of medical practice." In fact, if you really hate clinical medicine, medical management is not for you. It can be every bit as demanding and frustrating as clinical practice. Moreover, as the rate of change sweeping America's health care delivery system has accelerated, health care companies are reinventing themselves, developing competitive strategies that mean greater risk and more uncertainty than ever. Medical managers entering this brave new world, particularly those at the middle level, need to understand the landscape and be prepared to deal with it. The decision to be a manager should be a positive career choice, rather than one made by default. As the traditional separation of administrative and clinical matters is becoming obsolete, the modern physician manager must be a manager first and a clinician second. Bringing a clinical background to the new role of manager can certainly enrich the job, but it does not substitute for specific management skills and training. Whether medical management as such will ever become a recognized specialty is less important than the fact that only those who understand the language of both business and medicine will be able to straddle the various camps that now control the practice of medicine in this country.

For me, the career path from clinician to medical manager to CEO of a management search firm has been anything but straight. With each opportunity came a choice and a certain risk. But, in the end, it has been those forks in the road that have made all the difference.

References

1. de Llosa, P. "Executive Life: A New Twist in Consulting." *Fortune,* May 2, 1994, p. 84.

Chapter 13

Hospital Senior Vice President and Chief Medical Officer

by Peter L. Slavin, MD, MBA

Physician managers have the exciting opportunity to draw on their training in medicine and management to effect positive change in the delivery of health care services. Our health care system needs such individuals to bridge the cultural gulf between physicians and managers that often interferes with the performance of health care organizations.

Career Path

My career path has been guided by a long-standing interest in the practice of medicine and in the social and political issues that affect medical practice. While these intellectual interests have been a guide from the start of my career, serendipity has also played a major role in providing me with unexpected opportunities and insights into specific career steps.

At age 5, I developed staphylococcal pneumonia. I spent several days in the intensive care unit at Boston Children's Hospital. From that time on, I was fascinated by the wizardry of modern medical care and inspired by the work of the caring and capable physicians who treated me (especially my pediatrician, Albert Frank, MD).

My political interests are rooted in my family's active involvement in local Democratic politics. Early on, I learned the importance of being involved in community activities and advocating for key issues, such as adequate funding for the public school system.

As an undergraduate at Harvard College, I lived a somewhat schizophrenic life. As a biochemistry major and premedical student, I spent considerable time in science classes and the biochemistry labs. At the same time, I was actively involved in a student organization focused on political and public policy issues. I had no idea at that point how my interests in the practice of medicine and public policy would or could ever result in a career that combined those disciplines.

During the summer of my sophomore year, I volunteered in a local congressional campaign. My state representative, Ed Markey, whom I knew and respected from his previous campaigns, decided to run in a crowded Democratic primary for a vacant Massachusetts congressional seat. After a long but exhilarating campaign, he went on to win the Democratic primary and general election. I had the opportunity to work in his office the next summer in Washington, D.C., where he had been appointed to the Health Subcommittee of the Interstate Commerce Committee. That summer was one of the defining periods of my career. As I worked on such issues as national health insurance and the regulation of saccharine, I realized that my curiosity about medical practice and social issues could be combined in a career in health care policy.

Following my graduation from college, I took a year off before going to medical school. During that year, I worked in the Office of the Director (Donald Fredrickson, MD) of the National Institutes of Health. I became fascinated with various aspects of health research policy (e.g., the optimal balance between basic and clinical research funding) and learned more about the inner workings of Congress and the Executive Branch.

I returned to Boston to attend Harvard Medical School the following year. During the preclinical years, I was active in and led several policy-related student organizations. My years as a medical student were filled with many moving and stimulating patient encounters that reaffirmed my interest in and joy for the practice of medicine. I particularly enjoyed the rewarding longitudinal patient relationships experienced by general internists. I also found the science behind internal medicine particularly broad and challenging. For these reasons, I decided to apply for a residency in primary care/internal medicine and matched at Massachusetts General Hospital (MGH).

As my clinical skills grew as a resident, I became interested in the hospital systems and external resources that had such a dramatic impact on the health of my patients and on my ability to care for them well. I also saw that most of the extremely well-trained physicians with whom I worked and learned had little interest in or patience for these issues and also had little concern for overutilization of health care resources in their practices.

The same issues that stimulated me in Washington—the cost and quality of health care and access to it— suddenly came alive for me at MGH. It became apparent to me that the managers of this and other health care institutions made decisions about these issues on a daily basis and that these decisions had a very immediate and concrete impact on the delivery of health care. In addition, I sensed an enormous cultural gulf between physicians who were working hard to care for their patients and hospital managers who were doing their best to keep hospital programs working well and efficiently.

It dawned on me that a physician with an understanding of management might be able to play a very useful role in this setting. By understanding both medical and management issues, such individuals, I thought, might be able to identify opportunities to optimize the performance of the organization and the care it delivered to patients. Such physicians might also be able to bridge the cultural divide between physicians and managers by circulating and communicating comfortably in both camps.

During my senior residency, I had the good fortune of caring for a faculty member at a local business school who, after inquiring about my career interests, suggested that I attend business school. I initially dismissed this unconventional and impractical idea. A combined MD/MBA was almost unheard of at that time. Also, the thought of going back to school, with its associated actual and opportunity costs, seemed almost unthinkable.

After a year of work experience (a combination of clinical care, health services research, and management) at MGH following my residency, I decided to pursue a career in health care management. After a year of mulling over the suggestion of my patient that I go to business school, I decided to pursue this unusual suggestion. This decision was primarily motivated by my desire to be as well trained in management as I was in medicine.

My two years at Harvard Business School were intellectually exhilarating and eye opening. The intensity of the experience (particularly the first semester) was comparable to medical internship. My classmates were an especially bright and worldly group. The classroom experience was magical—a combination of hard-working, well-prepared students intersecting with an extremely capable and motivated faculty whose promotions were largely related to their teaching abilities. The subject matter (especially finance and operations management), although not taught in a health care context, was extremely applicable to the organization and management of health care. I also found the culture of business as powerful and captivating as the world of medicine.

As I approached graduation from business school, I was struck by the vast opportunities for physicians with this training in all sectors of the health care industry. After exploring opportunities in consulting, investment banking, and elsewhere, I ultimately decided to return to a health care delivery setting at Massachusetts General Hospital. This decision was motivated by my continued desire to practice medicine and by my intense interest in the management challenges close to the patient.

My work initially consisted of a combination of internal medicine practice, health services research, and hospital management. My management role was to develop from scratch a program to interest and involve physicians at MGH in cost and quality issues. This activity quickly mushroomed as the forces of managed care grew in the Boston marketplace. Many physicians within the hospital saw this program as an opportunity to shape their own destiny by optimizing the cost and demonstrating the quality of the services they delivered.

With a change in the leadership of the hospital in 1994, the new President, Samuel Thier, MD, asked me to become the Chief Medical Officer of the hospital.

Current Work

My current work as Senior Vice President and Chief Medical Officer of Massachusetts General Hospital and Medical Director of the Massachusetts General Physician Organization falls into several discrete activities:

Clinical Practice
I continue to practice and teach general internal medicine. I am scheduled to see patients one half day per week but am available to my patients for emergency or urgent problems at all times. I teach on the inpatient medical service during the month of July.

I also serve on the medical staff of the New England Patriots (National Football League) and New England Revolution (Major League Soccer). Because I am a life-long sports fan, this latter activity provides me with a fascinating behind the scenes view of professional athletics as well as some unusual medical challenges.

I continue to practice medicine almost entirely because I enjoy it immensely. I find that the challenges and the new developments in internal medicine are a constant source of intellectual excitement. In addition, relationships with patients, particularly those whom I have known for more than a decade, are more fulfilling personally than any other of my professional activities.

Practicing medicine also provides two benefits from a management perspective. First, it allows me a first-hand opportunity to see operational challenges and issues the medical staff faces in caring for inpatients and outpatients at MGH. Second, it brings me a degree of credibility with the medical staff not enjoyed by other managers, including nonpracticing physicians.

Reengineering

My most significant management responsibility at MGH is executive sponsorship of an institutionwide effort to redesign the way care is organized and delivered at the hospital. Operations Improvement (OI) was established more than a year ago to dramatically reduce MGH's operational costs and at the same time to improve the quality of service and care delivered to patients. The effort is organized into more than 20 multidisciplinary teams, some focused on hospital operations (e.g., clinical labs, patient care services, etc.) and others on clinical management issues (e.g., cardiac care, cancer care, etc.). Most of the leaders of these teams are well-respected physicians on the medical staff or senior managers of the MGH. At one point, the effort involved nearly 1,000 employees (more than 10 percent of the workforce).

The results of this effort, to date, have been quite satisfying. For example, multiple geographically scattered and semi-autonomous clinical labs have been consolidated into the core hospital labs, resulting in significant cost savings and service improvement to physicians and patients. On the clinical design side, more than 80 critical pathways have been developed, some resulting in dramatic decreases in length of stay and ancillary utilization. To date, cost per discharge has been reduced by 10 percent, and the bulk of the designed savings have not yet been implemented. More important than the expense savings to the hospital, in the long run, is the creation of a "learning organization" in multiple important parts of the institution.

Management of the effort requires numerous interrelated tasks on my part: (1) working with the President of MGH and the OI Director on a regular basis to guide the overall direction of the effort, (2) working with OI team leaders or other key institutional leaders on challenging political and substantive issues, and (3) organizing the infrastructure to support the effort (e.g., data systems, project management, communications strategy, etc.).

Professional Staff

As Chief Medical Officer of MGH, I am responsible for working with the chiefs of services on routine and more difficult professional staff issues. Specific tasks in this area include (1) responding to patient or employee complaints about the behavior or care of a physician and (2) determining the level of disciplinary action and external regulatory reporting warranted in specific situations.

Although this activity takes up a relatively small portion of my time, I view it as perhaps the most important activity in my portfolio. I believe that it is vital to treat employees fairly and to uphold vigilantly the values of the organization. In general, I do not believe hospitals and health care organizations have done an adequate job in the past of responding to substandard performance and conduct of professional staff members. Unless the medical profession takes these issues and responsibilities more seriously, we will see further external monitoring and management of physician behavior.

Medical Management

MGH (through Partners HealthCare System) has recently entered into several large, full-risk, commercial and Medicare capitated contracts that dramatically increase the importance of our medical management programs aimed at optimizing utilization for our patients covered under these contracts.

Medical management at MGH includes (1) case management, (2) information feedback to primary care physicians and specialists, (3) funds flow systems aimed at aligning incentives across all provider participants, (4) referral authorization systems, (5) establishment and management of numerous primary care and specialty medical management teams, (6) establishment of a high-quality, low-cost, nonacute service network (e.g., home care, subacute care, etc.), and (7) a pharmacy anti-detailing program promoting the prescribing of generic and other cost-effective drugs by our physicians.

Line Management

I have administrative responsibility for approximately 20 percent of the hospital's $600 million operating budget. The departments that report to me were chosen in part because their management intersects with some of my other responsibilities or because their cost structure (e.g., pathology) is largely driven by physician practice patterns. The departments currently reporting to me are:

● Clinical Care Management Unit

  ↪ Case Management
  ↪ Credentialing
  ↪ Payer Support
  ↪ Decision Support (supports Operations Improvement program)

- Social Services
- Pharmacy
- Radiology
- Pathology
- Office of Minority Health Professions
- Infection Control Unit

Career Advice

Career paths for physicians interested in management are designed like the streets of Boston—even if you know where you are going, it is not entirely clear how to get there. Until recently, physicians tended to get involved in management once they were winding down their careers in academics and/or clinical care. As management challenges in the health care industry have dramatically increased in complexity, so have the number of physicians interested early in their careers in pursuing career opportunities in management. This has been paralleled by a great supply of employment opportunities for physicians with such interests in all parts of the health care economy.

It seems to me that there are at least four ways for physicians interested in management to pursue such a career:

Just Do It

Some of the best physician managers I know have no formal management training. These individuals have a great natural knack for understanding the issues facing an organization and for articulating a clear strategy. They have typically worked their way up through the academic ranks and have demonstrated an ability to manage a complicated research program or an academic department. There are clearly physicians who can manage well without formal training. This is the exception rather than the rule and will become more difficult as health care management becomes increasingly complicated.

On the Job Training—Consulting

Management consulting provides physicians with an opportunity to work while learning a broad set of management issues. Many consulting firms are staffed with highly qualified MBAs who confer on junior members of the firm the benefits of their education. The project nature of consulting work provides physicians with an opportunity to be exposed to multiple management challenges over a relatively short period. Because the work of the consulting firm is to apply the knowledge of management disciplines to the client's situation, the physician consultant gets exposed to this process and, as a result, educated about many aspects of management. Several consulting firms with large health care practices and outstanding personnel (e.g., Boston Consulting Group, McKinsey & Co., and Bain & Co.) seem ideal for such training.

Master of Public Health (MPH)

Many schools of public health have departments of health policy and/or management and offer MPH degrees with a management focus. The strengths of these schools have, in the past, typically been in the disciplines necessary to understand the health problems of a population and to assess the impact of an intervention aimed at improving health (i.e., the fields of epidemiology, biostatistics, etc.). The management curriculum of these schools tends to be very health care-focused. The benefits of such a curriculum are that students learn a substantial amount about current management issues in health care. The curriculum of such programs tends to be more applied and less theoretical than can be found in more generic schools of management or business administration. These programs can also often be completed in one academic year, making them more practical than traditional MBA programs for physician trainees.

Master of Business Administration (MBA)

MBA programs offer future physician managers an opportunity to be exposed to a solid and comprehensive grounding in the management disciplines. In addition, these programs can expose physicians to faculty members and other students with interests in other industries; lessons from other industries can have enormous applicability in health care. MBA programs are available on a part-time or full-time basis, the latter taking 1.5 to 2 academic years to complete.

All of the management disciplines are applicable in a health care setting. Given my interests in health care delivery, I found finance and operations management the most relevant and useful in my management work to date. Training in finance allows a health care manager to structure a business decision and understand its financial consequences. Finance also proves useful in understanding the financial performance of an organization and in making sense out of financial statements.

Operations management is the science of business processes and is used by manufacturing firms worldwide to manage factory operations. Complicated health care delivery organizations can be analyzed with the tools and concepts of this science (e.g., cycle time etc.), as can the actual delivery of specific health care services (e.g., coronary artery bypass surgery). By using operations management, health care managers can streamline and improve the operations of health care institutions as well as the practice patterns of clinicians.

MBA training can provide physicians with solid management education as well as a credential that attests to their education. Many trainees considering this option are, however, concerned about the cost of MBA training, the commitment of time it requires, and the associated opportunity costs. As discussed in Chapter 2, several dual MD/MBA programs have recently been developed to address this problem.

Timing of Management Training

I frequently receive questions from medical students or other trainees about optimal timing for management training in the career of a physician. The range of possibilities is discussed in the introduction to this book. The answer to this question, in my view, rests in large part on the long-term career interests of the individual.

For physicians who are interested in practicing medicine or in the management of health care delivery, I strongly encourage deferment of management training until after residency training. By that career point, the physician's identity as a physician is firmly established and the trainee has significant experience in the clinical challenges of health care delivery. Both of these factors can help the young physician put the management training in some context. In addition, trainees who go directly from medical school to management training run the risk of never returning to residency training for a variety of reasons.

For physicians with interests in biotechnology or other aspects of the health care industry, I think the timing of management training is less critical. Under these circumstances, it would be appropriate to pursue management training immediately after medical school.

Conclusion

The current turmoil in the health care industry provides physicians with skills and interests in management with countless opportunities to effect badly needed improvements in the performance of health care organizations. By making their organizations more effective, physician managers can make a difference in the lives of patients.

There are many ways to get the training necessary to be successful in the field. Each individual should explore various options and tailor decisions to his or her interests and circumstances.

Combining a career as a physician and manager has been for me extremely stimulating and rewarding. A potential danger of such a career is the daily time commitment involved. Both medicine and management are full-time jobs; together they can be overwhelming. It is therefore critical to set limits early to avoid having one's personal life drowned out by professional activities.

My wife (Lori) and sons (Matthew and Daniel) are by far the greatest source of fulfillment in life. Everything that precedes this paragraph is simply icing on the cake.

Section III
The Physician Executive:
Regaining Control of Health Care

Chapter 14

The Emergence of the Physician CEO

By David J. Brailer, MD, PhD

Opportunities for physicians to become CEOs are more favorable than ever. Fundamental changes in the delivery of health care—financial risk being shifted to providers, care being integrated across sites, and clinical information being used as a means of achieving competitive success, to name a few—are offering a clear and perhaps one-time opportunity for physicians to take leading roles in shaping patient care at the system level. Physicians possess unique insights and skills that are crucial to the future success of the delivery system, so they are being sought as top-level leaders.

The emergence of the physician CEO is not a wholesale trend.[1,2] Many physicians are either unqualified for or disinterested in taking on such roles. However, it is the capstone of a systemwide change in the role of physicians in executive and leadership positions in the delivery system and is symbolic of the change under way in the health care industry. This chapter examines why physicians are being called on to become CEOs, the unique challenges physician CEOs face, and how physician executives can prepare for this role.

Market Drivers

As a result of today's managed care environment, purchasers are pressuring health care providers to reduce costs yet still maintain patient care at reasonable standards. At the same time, better informed consumers are increasingly demanding the highest quality patient care available. After more than a decade of unit cost reduction activities, health care delivery systems, knowing that the majority of discretionary costs are controlled by physicians,[3,4] have come to focus on the quantity of tests and therapies ordered for patients rather than on their cost. The ability to build strong physician relationships has become an important factor in their success as they organize to integrate care and manage financial risk.

To control clinical costs and quality without sacrificing physician relations, many providers are placing physicians in leadership positions, ranging from voluntary practicing physician leaders to part-time administrative physicians to full-time medical directors. As this occurs, many physicians are entering management positions that require them to exercise aspects of decision making and leadership they have not learned in full-time clinical practice and may not learn in their new physician executive positions, where managing "within the medical silo" deprives the executive of fundamental knowledge about core managerial techniques. This has brought about a resurgence of physicians' dreams—dormant since the 1930s—about being in control of patient care and has created a supply of trained physician executives who may be eligible to become CEOs.

Leadership Opportunity

The CEO of a health care delivery system—whether a hospital, a physician group, or an integrated health system—serves many roles in the organization. The manner in which the CEO leads the organization—as a leader, a change agent, a visionary, a cultural icon, a controller, a delegator, or a delineator—reflects the challenges the organization faces.[5] The best CEOs are versatile professionals who can exhibit many different styles of leadership, depending on what values and processes build core competence and competitive advantage for their organization at any point in time.[6] Very few CEOs, however, are so versatile that they can foresee and lead an organization through change when it transforms its fundamental business model and utterly rejects formerly held values and goals, as is happening in health care delivery today. Thus, in many cases, changing the CEO is itself part of an organization's process of growth.

Not surprisingly, the same fundamental market shift that has resulted in the emergence of clinical care management as a vital component of the delivery system is also dramatically changing expectations for the CEO. Across industries, market shifts induce changes in the culture, values, and operations of an organization, and a new type of CEO is symbolic of how the organization views itself and its role in the market.[7] This is true in health care as well. The chaotic market transition in health care delivery (e.g., rapid increases in managed care penetration) threatens the traditional revenue base and market role of the delivery system and the current leadership structure along with it. Chaos and fear are symptoms of the systematic process by which many years of assumptions about the market, about key relationships, and about the leaders themselves are being invalidated by these changes. In the few stable, mature markets in the United States in which delivery systems are gaining in strength, new assumptions, ideals, and cultures are taking hold as part of a new business model of health care delivery. This change is seen in sharp relief in the role of the CEO.

Looking forward, CEOs must understand how to organize and operate the health care delivery system as a clinical business. This means that the CEO must use physician relations, incentives, care protocols, clinical knowledge, and quality management just as readily as mergers, litigation, human resource management, cash flow, and market strategy. CEOs who understand the art and science of clinical care management can confer substantial and long-term competitive advantage on their organizations, provided they can also perform all of the requisite general management duties competently. These forces are the underlying drivers causing delivery systems to tap physicians as potential CEOs, positions for which they are often not prepared.

Management Challenges

The historical model of delivery system management has been described as administrators providing "rent-free workshops" to practicing physicians.[8] This model relied on the benevolence of administrators, the leverage of physicians, the agnosis of patients, and cost-plus payments. The predominant view of the delivery system was oriented toward a market strategy in the early 1980s and toward a financial and capital approach from the late 1980s to the present. Each of these orientations brought forth a well-trained cadre of executives and CEOs who personified its values within the delivery system. Indeed, in a late-1980s survey of delivery system CEOs, the ideal CEO was described as having strong skills in strategy formation and planning, finance, and negotiations and consensus building. Most CEOs then came from a finance or organizational development (e.g., consulting) background. A large share (22 percent) wanted increased education in finance. Many thought that CFOs were uniquely qualified to be CEOs of the future.[9]

Attitudes changed dramatically in the early 1990s. Reflecting the shift in perceptions about how best to respond to the threats faced by the delivery system, most of the respondents to a 1993 delivery system CEO survey believed that the number of physician CEOs would increase in the 1990s[10] (from a base of about 200 in 6,300 hospitals in 1996[11]). Financial management and market strategy, once sources of competitive advantage, are becoming competitive necessities. Accordingly, organizations can no longer differentiate themselves around these approaches. The new competitive advantage derives from the way in which physicians practice medicine, which is in the core competence of the physician executive.

The physician executive role is an expression of the collaborative relationship between management and physicians that is the basis for sophisticated clinical practice management. The emergence of the physician CEO is the next stage of development in the management of complex health care organizations. The principal challenge to physician executives who seek to become CEOs is developing new strengths—credibility among lay administrators and an ability to manage nonclinical aspects of the delivery system—to augment their preexisting strengths: respect among physicians and the ability to oversee clinical affairs.

The typical physician CEO today is 52 years old and male. Most are from primary care (44 percent) and about 90 percent are board-certified; nearly all spent a significant portion of their time in clinical practice prior to becoming CEOs.[10] These physicians entered management while still (part-time) practitioners. They had little formal training and experience in management and therefore sought out basic management education. Such a transition may not work well in the future. Because of growing practice responsibilities, physicians today face many barriers to seeking broad managerial responsibilities or training over extended periods. Those who are able to adapt their practices are being paid a management salary equal to their lost practice income, which is much higher than the salary of an equivalent manager. As a result, there are substantial income barriers to their making an executive transition. CEOs may earn more than physicians, but generally only after several years of significantly lower income as full-time managers.

The most likely modern cohort of potential CEOs is full-time medical directors (also called chief medical officers or vice presidents of medical affairs). This group has extensive medical management experience and is usually well educated about management. However, many physicians in this category spend most, if not all, of their time managing the affairs of other physicians and have little experience in financial, strategic, human resources, and other areas outside of medicine. There is a small subset of full-time physician executives who have gained extensive managerial education and experience and are seeking positions outside medical management where they can sharpen their reasoning, leadership, and strategic skills alongside similarly skilled peers. It is this small subset that is most likely to supply the CEOs of the next millennium.

Unique Role

Physician executives have become widely accepted in the managed care market as essential supervisors of practicing physicians. They review key hospitalization and treatment decisions made by practicing physicians to ensure that cost-effective therapies are being followed. They manage by enabling physicians to comply with often strict clinical protocols and measure their effectiveness in terms of medical loss reductions (lower payments out of premiums). Providers now find themselves in need of physician executives, as managed care organizations shift risk to providers. Because delivery systems face economic pressure to become more efficient and the greatest potential source of efficiency improvement is in the clinical arena, development and inclusion of physician executives is vital to the success of integrated delivery systems.[12]

Historically, management of the delivery system has been overseen by nonclinicians, with physicians in supporting roles. Physician executives, however, having had direct responsibility for the health of patients and of populations, possess the skills to manage the organization when clinical decision making is the primary determinant of competitive survival. They can decentralize much of the decision making and initiative to practicing physicians and engage in a collaborative dialogue that promotes loyalty to the delivery system. Physician executives will encounter fewer of the problems experienced by traditional managers in organizational governance. The major problems in physician practice management identified by Megel et al.,[13] for example, included a perceived resistance from physicians, the lack of authority to mandate action, and the conflict between physicians and management. These tensions are eased for physician executives who have gained credibility with their peers by virtue of their clinical experience and who can then initiate a significant change in practice patterns.

By addressing the concerns of staff physicians in addition to those of the purchaser and the consumer, physician executives can dramatically improve the quality and efficiency of clinical practice.[14] Staff physicians are not readily susceptible to managerial oversight by nonphysicians, who may be perceived as cost-cutting threats to physician autonomy. Physician CEOs acknowledge that management of patient care must occur within a clinically relevant framework, which appeals to the staff physician's ultimate concern for the patient.[15] Physician executives are a powerful means of creating sustainable change in integrated delivery systems and of placing physicians in the position to lead others in making change.[16] The physician CEO with good management training not only can uniquely understand the importance of these issues—often from personal experience in practice—but also can incorporate these views into the culture and operations of the delivery system.

Skill Development

CEOs across firms in all industries have much in common. Manufacturing and service firms outside health care seek CEOs with several essential qualities: strategic vision, operating experience, leadership and team building skills, performance-driven personality, logical judgment mixed with prudent risk-taking, financial acumen, credibility and values, technical knowledge, communication skills, and ability to make change.[17,18] These qualities are relevant to delivery system CEOs,[5] although they are more well established in other industries than in health care, where the CEO was considered an "administrator" until the late 1970s.[19]

Because health care has only recently developed an industrial base and infrastructure, delivery system CEOs have sought knowledge about health care delivery management from outside health care. This technology transfer has provided many new ideas to delivery systems that were developed in other industries, such as customer satisfaction or market planning. Recent technology transfer of ideas from other service industries to managed care organizations, including call centers for demand management or information vehicles to bypass traditional market geography (e.g., teleradiology), have rapidly become disseminated within the health care market. Notably, most concepts adopted from other industries have little relationship to the manner in which patient care is delivered, but focus on how the delivery system organizes itself.

Changes currently under way in health care require deep understanding of how patient care works and how it can be improved. Hence, much less can be learned from other industries that will benefit this unique aspect of the delivery system. It is difficult to learn how to care for a diabetic, for example, from other industries. This is one reason why physician CEOs are sought. They bring a deep insight about the core production processes of patient care and knowledge of how the profession of medicine can be harnessed as a competitive apparatus. Their challenge is to gain basic management skills and internalize general leadership characteristics, as well as to assimilate their knowledge across business and medicine into a cohesive "management theory."

Issues surrounding the emergence of the physician CEO are being investigated at The Wharton School at the University of Pennsylvania. The Wharton School has a 25-year history of health care management programs and has produced a large number of skilled and respected leaders in the health care industry. Wharton has had one of the longest standing and largest programs for education of physician executives, including MBA and PhD programs, fellowships, information dissemination through the Internet and information technology, faculty-sponsored research initiatives, executive education, and interactive learning through seminars and conferences sponsored by The Wharton School in conjunction with the Leonard Davis Institute and the School of Medicine at the University of Pennsylvania.

A recent Clinical Performance Improvement Roundtable and Case Study Session at The Wharton School brought together about 50 chief medical officers from large physician groups, clinics, academic medical centers, and integrated delivery systems across the United States. The group identified 10 skill areas of high importance to the development of physician CEOs. In descending order of importance, these areas were physician leadership development, clinical performance improvement methods, operations and program implementation, information systems, mergers and delivery system integration, outcomes and quality measurement, financial analysis and economic measurement, disease management, law and ethics, and medical management techniques.

To understand how this group develops management skills, participants were asked to identify sources of education and development for the skills. They cited many teaching sources and on-the-job experiences for learning medical management (tenth ranked). "Medical management" includes utilization review, physician credentialing, guideline development, and physician payment, the core aspects of managing physicians. Few participants, however, could identify sources of education or job experience for the other nine skill areas. Of particular concern were leadership development and nonclinical management (e.g., finance, information systems, etc.), areas they deemed important to a CEO's ability to manage and in which they identified their largest weaknesses. The Wharton School is currently developing fellowships that seek to broaden the top-level skills and experiences of these physicians.

Conclusion

Rapid changes in the health care marketplace have elevated the management of clinical affairs to paramount importance. This has created irresistible demand for senior-level physicians to become CEOs of multibillion-dollar delivery systems. In order to take advantage of the leadership opportunity opened up by these fundamental market changes and to be successful as CEOs, physician executives need education and experience to broaden their knowledge beyond the management of clinical affairs. This training cannot be gained while in the CEO seat without substantial distraction (from time spent learning) and risk (from intolerable mistakes), so all physician executives—whether or not they see a CEO position in their immediate future—need to seek out activities that increase their senior management skills, insights, and experiences.

Physician executives can do many things to enhance their top-level management skills and prepare themselves to become CEOs. First, a perspective beyond the medical management silo must be achieved. While it is important to know how to deal with physicians in practice and to supervise clinical decision making, there are many other aspects of the delivery system that must be mastered, ranging from finance to operations to legal affairs to marketing. Excellence in medical management is a unique physician executive skill, but it is not a substitute for general management abilities.

Second, credibility with traditional lay executives must be earned. While some lay executives may flatly reject physicians as leaders without regard for their abilities, many observe that physician executives are unrealistic and naïve about nonclinical affairs. Learning these areas of health care delivery will take substantial classroom and field experiences in settings in which mistakes can be made without dire consequences. The willingness to learn this aspect of management would in itself be an important means of gaining respect from lay colleagues.

Third, reasoned judgment skills must be learned. In their core development, physicians learn to avoid risk and to ignore resource constraints. This does not provide the best training for senior managerial decision making, the essence of which is managing risk—taking necessary risks, defining risk and benefit, and choosing a course of action despite uncontrollable risk—and managing constrained resources—budgeting, prioritizing, and making difficult trade-offs.

Fourth, credibility with physicians must be maintained. It is no surprise that most physician CEOs are board-certified and spent some time in practice, as these experiences shape their ability to bring the physician's perspective to managerial decisions.

Rudolph Virchow may have had today's physician CEO in mind when, in the mid-1800s, he wrote, "...if medicine is the science of the healthy as well as of the ill human being (as it ought to be), what other science is better suited to propose laws as the basis of the social structure...."[20] In many ways, Virchow's challenge can be simply restated as: Physicians ought to be delivery system leaders, and if they do not take this challenge, they should accept the governance, values, and priorities of others who will lead. To the extent that the restructured health care delivery market will be durable over many years, this may be the last chance for physicians to shape and mold the care of patients and the disposition of medical practice on a widespread basis.

References

1. LeTourneau, B., and Curry, W. "Physicians as Executives: Boon or Boondoggle." *Frontiers of Health Services Management* 13(3):3-25, Spring 1997.

2. LeTourneau, B., and Curry, W. "Do Physician Executives Make a Difference? Reply." *Frontiers of Health Services Management* 13(3):43-5, Spring 1997.

3. Levit, K., and others. "Health Care Spending in 1994: Slowest in Decades." *Health Affairs* 15(2):130-144, Summer 1996. Also Health Care Financing Administration, Office of the Actuary, data from the Office of National Health Statistics.

4. Rakich, J. *Managing Health Services Organizations*. Philadelphia, Pa.: W.B. Saunders, 1985.

5. Kent, T., and others. "Leadership in the Formation of New Health Care Environments." *Health Care Supervisor* 15(2):27-34, Dec. 1996.

6. Farkas, C., and Wetlaufer, S. "The Way Chief Executive Officers Lead." *Harvard Business Review* 74(3):110-22, May-June 1996.

7. Gifford, D. "CEO Turnover: The Importance of Symbolism." *Harvard Business Review* 75(1):9-10, Jan.-Feb. 1997.

8. Pauly, M. *Doctors and Their Workshops*. Chicago, Ill.: University of Chicago Press, 1980.

9. Eubanks, P. "The New Hospital CEO: Many Paths to the Top." *Hospitals* 64(23):26-31, Dec. 5, 1990.

10. Sherer, J. "Physician CEOs: Ranks Continue to Grow." *Hospitals* 67(9):42, May 5, 1993.

11. *AHA Guide to the Health Care Field*. Chicago, Ill.: American Hospital Association, 1996.

12. Brailer, D. "Report on the Wharton Study Group on Clinical Performance Improvement." *Journal of Clinical Outcomes Management* 4(5):37-43, Sept.-Oct. 1997.

13. Megel, M., and others. "Conflicts Experienced by QAI Professionals: A Delphi Study." *Journal of Nursing Care Quality* 10(2):75-82, Jan. 1996.

14. Greco, P., and Eisenberg, J. "Changing Physicians' Practices." *New England Journal of Medicine* 329(17):1271-4, Oct. 21, 1993.

15. Gates, P. "Clinical Quality Improvement: Getting Physicians Involved." *Quality Review Bulletin* 19(2):56-61, Feb. 1993.

16. Brailer, D. "The Public Spirited Physician." In *Future Practice Alternatives in Medicine*, 2nd edition, Nash, D., Editor. Chicago, Ill.: Igaku Shoin Medical Publishers, 1993.

17. Neff, T. Top 12 Traits of Today's CEOs." *Chief Executive Magazine* (108):38-9, Nov. 1995.

18. Callen, J. "Critical Skills and the CEO." *Chief Executive Magazine* (84):34-7, April 1993.

19. Neuhauser, D. *Coming of Age: A 50-Year History of the American College of Hospital Administrators and the Profession It Serves*, 1933-1983. Chicago, Ill.: American College of Hospital Administrators, 1983.

20. Virchow, R. *Disease, Life and Man*, Rather, L., Translator. New York, N.Y.: Collier Books, 1962.

Chapter 15

The Career Marketplace for Physician Executives

by John S. Lloyd, MBA, MPH

The health care job market today is truly wide open for excellent physician executives. Opportunities abound in health care systems, corporate offices of pharmaceutical firms and insurance companies, information systems firms, outcomes management and practice management entities, universities and medical schools—even, or perhaps especially, in hospitals. An executive with vision and the leadership ability to get the job done can go all the way to the top.

Having ability both as a physician and an executive certainly affords distinct advantages in the competition for the best jobs in the health care arena; this is an ideal time for physician executives to exploit their unique blend of skills and experience. A physician could be named head of General Motors or General Electric—or even, if one were willing to endure the rigors of a national campaign, President of the United States. William Frist, MD, is already a member of the U.S. Senate, and we will watch his career. Of course, no real or imaginary bar ever prevented physicians from rising to these heights; what is new is the experienced cadre of physician executives. We only wish there were more who were ready to take advantage of these challenges and opportunities.

Those of us who can recall earlier times know that the evolution of physician executives—from modest beginnings as medical directors to today's superstar executives—was achieved in a generation. In about 20 years, we have seen a slow, steady increase in the numbers of talented people who are both physicians and executives in leadership positions in virtually every type of health care organization. Private hospitals, public multihospital corporations, managed care companies, insurance firms, universities, and government agencies are all today headed by physician executives.

What special mix of traits and abilities has transformed some physicians into the kind of hard-charging executives who are ideally suited to take on senior roles in all sorts of organizational configurations and structures? Some are, as Shakespeare noted long ago, "born great; some achieve greatness; and some have greatness thrust upon them." Into that latter category of greatness we could easily insert the earliest physicians in management. Many did not choose the work; it chose them.

First: a Need for Managers

Physicians in general in the late '70s and early '80s were neither trained for nor psychologically suited to roles as managers. Doctors customarily saw themselves as solo practitioners, not team players. As professionals, they were often unwilling to confront other physicians on any subject more controversial than how many strokes had been taken on the eighth hole.

Transition: DRGs Widen the Gap

However, with the introduction of DRGs, the essentially passive role of hospital medical director (e.g., keeping committee minutes, updating Joint Commission information, and ensuring the credentialing process worked smoothly) became much more active. Health care organizations were compelled to examine closely—and, often, to reform—their methods of doing business. Knowing and managing costs were more important than ever to providers of high-quality care, and both hospitals and managed care organizations needed clinical input to survive.

The need was clear: Managers who understood and could speak the language of the medical process had to be found. And where better to find them than in the organization's own group of physicians? Their clinical backgrounds and personal relationships with other physicians gave them an edge in the competition for emerging roles as managers.

For the first time, many physicians actually had direct oversight of decisions of their peers. Although still largely seen as clinical matters, the decisions had an obvious financial impact on physicians and on the institution as well. When the hospital or system sought to develop a PPO or similar bridge structure with physicians, physician leaders again were called on to manage the people and the process. And, once the doors to health care's executive suite were opened to real management opportunities for physicians, a trickle and then a flood of enthusiastic, energetic individuals began to raise their own management profiles.

Howard Grant, MD, JD, set out to make an executive career from his management roles. Now CEO at Shriners Temple Children's Hospital, Philadelphia, Pennsylvania, he was once a senior pediatric resident working in a hospital's medical records department. He saved the hospital an estimated $400,000 by developing systems to identify and correct miscoded charts. Howard had a considerable interest in management, which he has since extended into a notable executive career. He commented recently to me, reflecting on his executive position: "This is a much tougher job than I thought it would be." Well, he has been challenged but not overwhelmed.

Elliot Sussman, MD, President of Lehigh Valley Medical Center in Allentown, Pennsylvania, is another physician executive who chose his path through management early, building jobs where none had existed previously. Dr. Sussman was a Harvard-trained internist when he took on his first management roles at the University of Pennsylvania and then the University of Chicago.

Not everyone can do what those two did, but the right opportunities and a little bit of luck might be all you need to get started.

Physician Executives Gain Prominence

The physician-in-management era, prompted by DRGs and the managed care revolution, made many physicians take a new look at their chosen career field of medicine. Some physicians eventually opted out of medicine entirely; others took themselves back to school for MBAs or other management degrees and then found management roles—inside or outside of health care. Ultimately, the emergence of integrated delivery networks/systems (IDN/IDS) offered real scope to physicians who were ready to move from management into true executive roles.

It is my business, as an executive search consultant who follows trends, to know the individuals who blaze the trails. For example, I recall when Wynn Presson (not a physician) was CEO at Swedish American Hospital in Rockford, Illinois. Wynn groomed the extraordinary Bob Henry, a psychiatrist, for management at the hospital. When Wynn left in the early '80s, the board named Bob Henry CEO, and he, in turn, mentored another physician executive, Bob Klint, who succeeded him in the CEO position.

That was back in the days (just 10 or 12 years ago) when you could have held an ACPE national meeting in a small conference room. There may have been 1,000 members then; today there are over 12,000, and growing! It was about that time that the MBA and other management degrees (MHA, MPH, MIS, etc.) began to be perceived by physicians as professional tickets to a management career.

They have learned that merely having a ticket is not enough. In a long-ago Woody Allen movie, a college instructor says she must leave "to teach class." Intentionally misunderstanding her to make a point, another character sneers: "You can't teach class. You've either got it or you don't. But you can't teach it." Similarly, physicians in management have learned they cannot just assume executive status; it requires more than good will, a management degree, and a desire to serve. Only in the past few years can we claim that a real "pool" of physician executives has developed.

Most physicians do not become executives unless an organization needs them for that work. Individuals rarely nominate themselves; usually, one must be asked, because of a special blend of skills and talents. For example, two of the premier cancer treatment facilities in the world—Memorial Sloan-Kettering in New York and M.D. Anderson Center in Houston—have identified charismatic physician executives to be their CEOs. John Mendelsohn, MD, and Paul Marks, MD, are visionaries who bring a powerful inspirational purpose to the struggle for cancer cures. Their organizations are confident they chose the right men for those jobs largely because of their visions for victory over cancer.

Or consider William Kelly, MD, Executive Vice President at the University of Pennsylvania Hospital Medical Center and Dean of the University of Pennsylvania School of Medicine, who has the hospital, the faculty practice, managed care, and the medical school reporting to him. When Dr. Kelly asked the trustees to help him redefine the University of Pennsylvania within the new health care environment, they gave him an enthusiastic go-ahead—backing him in the $300 million purchase of medical practices and the formation of a primary-care feeder network throughout the Delaware Valley. Michael Johns, MD, Vice President of Health Affairs at Emory University, has a somewhat similar role at his academic institution.

Exceptions do exist, however. David Skinner, MD, literally walked out of the surgical suite into the President/CEO role at New York Cornell Medical Center. He still regularly does surgery. Another exception to the rule that comes to mind is Michael Maves, MD, MBA, an otolaryngologist who is Executive Director of his professional society. He has consciously prepared himself for an executive role by keenly studying other executives to learn what others do to succeed. The common thread in every case is that the board to whom the physician executive reports is open to change, ready to accept and work with new concepts. They have rejected the old-fashioned perception that all physicians are bad business people. They are ready to be inspired.

Part Iaccoca, Part Welby

When a Detroit automobile company board decides it needs an outstanding marketing executive to be CEO, it selects such an executive. And in the business pages, we read every day of yet another executive hired to downsize an organization into profitability and improved return on equity. But there are no guarantees. When a corporation decides it needs another strategic emphasis—international trade instead of cost-cutting, for example—another new executive will be hired to meet that new need. And the former executive usually takes early retirement.

Similarly, a health care organization with medical staff problems could do worse than to choose a physician executive—a leading community citizen—as its CEO to instill trust and confidence. But today that physician must be more than a kindly figurehead. Boards today expect an MD/MBA to combine the hard-nosed business acumen of a Lee Iaccoca with the nurturing medical style of a Dr. Marcus Welby. The remarkable thing is that so many physician executives actually carry it off.

Look at David Kessler, MD, who served in the position of Commissioner of the Food and Drug Administration under two presidents. When I first met David, he was a young emergency physician who became Medical Director at Montefiore Hospital in the Bronx. Later, at the FDA, he oversaw many of the key decisions of the day: product packaging, food nutrition labeling, the introduction of no-fat foods, the decline of smoking advertising, and the first serious consideration of nicotine as a drug, AIDS drugs that seem to be effective, and so much more. He was the right person for the times and the place.

Or consider Samuel R. Nussbaum, MD, who is Executive Vice President, Medical Affairs, at the BJC system in St. Louis, Missouri. A faculty member at Harvard Medical School, he went to Blue Cross of Massachusetts as the person responsible for relations with physicians and groups and then was recruited by a provider to develop a network of physicians. He managed physicians throughout his career but has never managed a hospital. His role now is essentially marketing BJC's provider services to physicians in Missouri and western Illinois, and he understands the concerns of physicians better than almost anyone else, in the view of the board and BJC senior executives.

Essential Executive Skills

When an organization hires our executive search firm to assist in identifying the right individual for an open position, the customary first step is to develop with it a list of job specifications. The job "specs" are the blueprint used to complete the rest of the search. When it knows what the client wants accomplished, the consultant team can go out to find people who can do those defined tasks. Job "specs" are then used in interviews by savvy boards to help them evaluate how well their stated needs will be met by candidates.

In almost every CEO search engagement we have undertaken in the past five years or more, our client organizations say these are the key skills and traits they want a CEO to possess, in abundance:

- **Vision.** An executive sees the future for the organization and can pull the various parts and pieces (and people) of the organization into a cohesive whole.

- **Communication.** An executive can share that vision with others and is able to motivate employees and community groups. Communication also involves infusing spirit and purpose into doing one's daily job. And, by listening to all the constituencies who must be heard, an executive can achieve consensus.

- **Drive for Excellence.** An executive seeks excellence in others and is able to identify and nurture others' executive talents. The level of expectation is high, and outcomes usually match up.

- **Strategic Thinking.** An executive knows there are many paths and is willing to ask directions for all of them. Comfort with information systems allows executives to make informed judgments.

- **Financial Acumen.** An executive is more than a theorist or a figurehead. At the end of the day, the books have to balance and the overall financial picture must be a healthy one for true executive success.

- **Physician Relations**. While it might seem to be a given, it cannot be assumed that a physician executive will be particularly skilled in this area. Indeed, as some have found out rather painfully, their physician relations may only be good at a place where they are already well-known. Physician relations must be a portable skill.

Are You Ready for a Physician Executive Career?

Recently, a critical mass has been achieved in some institutions: At least one member of the senior management group is a physician executive. That is important, because, when a CEO position becomes available, boards often want to look at internal candidates before they open their search to the larger universe of qualified individuals. If a physician executive is on the scene, with credentials and relationships in good order, he or she is much more likely to be selected as CEO.

In our recent experience as a search firm, when a senior position (CEO, Senior Vice President, etc.) has opened at an integrated delivery system/network, the board generally wants continuity and seeks new leadership from inside rather than from outside. And, in many cases, there is a physician executive poised and ready to accept the challenge.

The newest opportunities for physician executives are in information systems, whether for a data management company such as HCIA, Inc., or with NCQA (National Committee for Quality Assurance), or like Mitchell Morris, MD, director of information systems at M.D. Anderson Cancer Center. He uses information technology to make better diagnoses for cancer treatment. Another example is David Blumenthal, MD, who runs the Harvard information center and also sees patients two days a week. Brent James, MD, a physician with Intermountain Healthcare who uses computers to analyze clinical information, is another classic instance.

An Identity Crisis of Sorts

Some physicians fear they will lose their identities as physicians if they become executives. That is a reasonable concern, as the priorities, tempo, and pace of the two jobs are very different. But the rewards—financial and emotional—are also very real and can be attractive enough to loosen the firm hold on a physician identity. When Witt/Kieffer recently asked physician executives nationwide to consider their different roles and rank them, 80 percent said that, five years ago, they thought of themselves first as physicians; only 13 percent thought of themselves first as leaders. Today, only 42 percent of the same group say they are physicians first; more (47 percent) see themselves first as leaders. This is a startling metamorphosis. If a physician executive finds that fact to be intolerable, then, as the old saying goes: "If you didn't want to go to Minneapolis, why did you get on the train?"

You can walk on the edge for a time but, sooner or later, as you pursue an executive/managerial career, you will have to choose on which side to come down. Here are some things you should think about long and hard before that happens. If you are considering taking on a management or executive role, be aware of these key issues:

- **Mobility.** Executives base their careers on being willing to go where the best opportunities exist. Those who will not make career moves are not very successful. But physicians generally like to put down roots, to remain in a place where they are known and respected. They do not hop around every few years, as executives do. Experience has shown that most physicians remain within 500 miles of their residency. Are you more mobile than that?

- **Popularity.** Executives can tolerate not being liked by everyone, as part of their job. But physicians, largely, like to be thought well of and appreciated. It can be considered one of the rewards for the long hours and anguish they see every day. In contrast, being disliked (if not actively loathed) by a number of people is part of the executive's job.

- **Different Type of Compensation.** The average senior executive's earning power is not so different from the average physician's, but the compensation method is. In medicine, you are compensated directly, for the work you have done today. "An honest day's work for a day's pay" is a concept that appeals to many people. However, in management or as an executive, your compensation rewards are often much more long-term. Your salary may be set-up to increase over a period of years, or you may be offered incentives that depend on measures at one-, three-, or even five-year intervals. You may have a percentage of your income tied to the success of the risks you took. Even more frequently, your pay may depend on the performance of many other people totally outside of your control.

- **Different type of stress.** Most physicians feel they know all about job stress; they make life-and-death decisions daily. Yet many physicians have never had to deal, as executives do, with a lengthy, administrative decision-making process, one in which people must be influenced and persuaded. For physicians, the key decision is in the diagnosis. Once they diagnose correctly, they can select the optimal treatment. In management, the solutions often are multiple. There is no one right answer. The physician in management has to become comfortable with ambiguity, to be able to accept the stress of knowing that no snap diagnosis will solve things. Physicians in management often say they think decisions "never get made." They mean the pace is glacial compared to what they are accustomed to as practicing physicians. And that causes stress.

Importance of a Mentor

For physician executives, the management mentor role is still fairly new. In a 1996 national survey of physician executives conducted by Witt/Kieffer, respondents said their mentors provide awareness of educational, training and management opportunities. In addition, mentors lead by example and provide management/leadership modeling and demonstrations of management techniques. Some mentors give direction and advice on organizational thinking. Other mentors offer counsel on professional development, including management and leadership skills, personal experience and professional growth. And mentors offer general encouragement, guidance, support, good listening, and feedback.

Overall, 42 percent of physician executive respondents said a mentor "played a pivotal role" in their executive careers. Those in payers (insurance and managed care companies) were a bit more likely (46 percent) than those in providers such as hospitals and systems (40 percent) to have had a mentor. Their mentors are senior health care executives (75 percent) or colleagues at the same level (16 percent). Non-health care executives or others are 9 percent. Most mentors (74 percent) are themselves physician executives. Those who were mentored reported mentoring others in turn—in payers (63 percent) and in providers (66 percent).

What Does It Take to Get to the Top?

I have retitled a presentation I used to give to physician groups on "How to Become a CEO." Increasingly, today's physician executives have less interest in the top job and more in senior vice president roles. But whether you want to rise to CEO or are aiming a little lower, to develop your management roles into a true executive career, I offer the schematic below (with apologies, of course, to Dr. Maslow) as a guide. To achieve a position of leadership, you must begin with basic skills and enhance your career profile accordingly.

Lloyd's Pyramid of Health Care Leadership Attainment

Leadership

Create organizational vision

Increased management responsibility

Work with a mentor

Management experience

Basic skills

While only you can decide whether to take the steps outlined here, this is clearly what the marketplace expects of you for success.

Chapter 16

Physician CEOs: Breaking the Glass Ceiling

by Jennifer R. Grebenschikoff

One of the top positions in medical management for physician executives is chief executive officer. It is also one of the most difficult to break into because of the traditional preference for nonphysicians with business training and background. But many physician executives are breaking the glass ceiling because they are proving that their clinical background gives them a valuable added perspective in utilization, quality, and cost issues. Also, through training seminars, advanced degrees, and on-the-job training, they bring business skills to the table that rival those of nonphysicians.

Hiring physician executives as health care CEOs makes perfect sense, says Ed Lowenstein, MD, CEO of Physician Associates of Florida, Maitland, because, "The head of a blacksmith shop ought to be a blacksmith. The head of an accounting firm ought to be an accountant."

Physician executives who pursue this powerful position do so for the challenge and for the impact they can make on the health of their communities. Some may say that physician CEOs are "regaining control" of health care. But, because "control" means being in a position to affect how health care is delivered, I am not sure physician executives have ever lost control. By moving into senior management positions and preparing themselves to become CEOs, they are ensuring that the community will benefit from their commitment, and they are helping the profession of medicine to maintain its "control" of the business of health care.

Every physician executive who has made it to the top has taken virtually the same road, but how they traveled down that road and how long it took them to arrive is an individual experience. I selected six physicians currently in CEO positions and asked them to share their road maps.

Ed Lowenstein, MD
CEO, Physician Associates of Florida
Maitland, Florida

Ed Lowenstein learned management at an early age. His dad, who ran a large electrical engineering firm, engaged him in discussions about management style and technique and about how to get people to perform on the job. His interest in management was rekindled while he was in a private pediatrics practice in Atlantic City,

N.J., when a group of local physicians began meeting to form an independent practice association (IPA).

"They wanted young turks like me to get involved in peer review and case management and financial stuff, and come to meetings every Monday night," he recalled. "For five or six years, I gave my evenings helping the IPA. I got to know some of the people, so when Prudential was doing its group model development back in the early '80s, it asked me to come down and start a group model in Orlando. The rest of it is history."

Lowenstein started the group as a medical director 13 years ago. Three years ago, he was promoted to CEO. "The people (physicians) who do this work need to expand their minds. The decisions you have to make and the way you have to conduct yourself and how you think about problem-solving expands way beyond what you do as a physician," Lowenstein says. He believes the best way to advance to CEO is "working in management roles and coming up through the ranks. I think it's 80 percent on-the-job training, and about 20 percent is going to courses and learning a little about finance, law, and some technical skills." However, he stresses that CEOs do not have to be experts in every aspect and that, if they put good teams together, the expertise comes from them and the leadership comes from the CEO.

Lowenstein's advice to those who wish to become CEOs is to "chair some committees dealing with the tough issues, be head of a clinical department, work on some political issues, and learn how to do some budgeting. Move through it on a small scale and gradually enlarge the scale."

Read, network, take courses, and find a mentor. "Together it yields a decent manager in 10 years." Lowenstein encourages risk-taking, shedding skepticism, and moving ahead on vision.

Lowenstein does not have a master's degree and does not believe physicians need one to become CEOs. "Docs look at MBAs as a ticket," he says. "They think they just turn in their ticket and get a management job. And that's where I think the paradigm falls apart. If somebody came with an MBA and no experience, and somebody came with management experience and no MBA, it would be a hands-down choice for the latter."

As health care continues to evolve and change, Lowenstein predicts that many new senior management positions will open. "Medical groups will consolidate, and, through consolidation, there will be larger groups of physicians working together. They will need a management team to lead them, and, typically, they will want a physician to head the management team."

Robert A. Catalano, MD, MBA
CEO, Olean Community Hospital
Olean, NY

Catalano was first hired as medical director of his 217-bed community hospital. When the CEO retired three years later, he was promoted to CEO at age 37. "An MBA was necessary to get into the door," he says. "Several board members subsequently told me that I would have never been selected as CEO had I not had my MBA. I was surprised to hear that, but most of our board members are business people, and I suspect that may be true of many boards. They like to talk to people they feel are similar to them. They equate someone with an MBA as a sound business person."

Although an MBA was a requirement of the job, Catalano says he had other skills that are not taught in college that he considers more important than the degree. "The irony of the comment made by the board members is that I do believe the majority of skills I had preceded the MBA, and the MBA was not the most important thing to bring to the table. The interpersonal skills were more important, dealing with difficult situations, change—that's probably more important," he says.

Catalano acquired an MBA at age 33 while serving as medical director. After acting as administrator of the department of ophthalmology at an academic medical center and dealing with capital budgets and operating budgets, he decided he needed a rapid way to acquire the knowledge he needed.

Why did he want to become a CEO? Catalano says there were two reasons: first, because he thought he could do a good job and, second, because he saw ways to improve health care for the community and ways to accomplish things for the hospital, the medical staff, and the hospital staff.

"I didn't want to control anybody," he says. "The CEO has to look at things in terms of the community as opposed to one segment of the community—the medical staff. So, if physicians are thinking of being hospital administrators so they can make things more comfortable for physicians, they are losing sight of the bigger picture. The bigger picture is: what's best for the community. If you want to be a CEO, you have to do it for the right reasons." In fact, decisions CEOs must make often run counter to the agendas of physicians in the organization, he adds.

The CEO position differs from the medical director position in that more contracting work and more legal knowledge are necessary to do the job, he says. But the bulk of the skills mirror those of a successful medical director: interpersonal skills, problem-solving, decision-making, personal traits that are not in the curriculum of any college and cannot be learned on the job.

Eugene McDannald, MD, MBA
Executive Director Asante Health
Warner Robins, Georgia

McDannald left a private anesthesiology practice to take a position as CEO of a medical products company. He had served as a medical director and department chair of anesthesia at an academic medical center and as medical director at a smaller hospital, where he eventually ran every department. But the experience was not adequate preparation for the CEO role. Although he managed to function, he relied heavily on his subordinates and spent two very uncomfortable years feeling guilty that he was not more prepared for the job.

At age 57, he decided to pursue an MBA. "I felt that if I was going to progress, I needed to go forward," says McDannald. "If I was going to stay on the administrative side, I needed the tools, the skill sets, the information, and I needed to know the thinking of other people who were my peers. I needed to have the same thought processes."

McDannald went through the MBA program at University of Colorado, which he selected because of the quality of its faculty, while he was working full time and found it to be more challenging than he expected. "It's a time-consuming, family-threatening, leisure time-ruining process," he recalls. "You've got to say, 'I'm dedicated to doing it. I'm going to do it. Here's the way I'm going to do it.' Failing to have all those commitments, you will not succeed."

But do not expect to land a senior management position just because you have an MBA, he warns. "A friend of mine from the graduate program is just absolutely mad at the world because nobody has offered him a job he thinks he's worthy of," says McDannald. "But the ticket is not the answer. In medical administration, it's also having gone through some of the hard knocks that other medical administrators go through. I've been an operating officer for a hospital. I did that because I needed to know the ins and outs of how a hospital runs," he adds.

McDannald says the MBA program gave him the tools he needed to succeed in the CEO position: health care financing, medical information systems, systems thinking, problem-solving, personnel relations. "I think we're going to see more physicians with MBAs," says McDannald. "I think that those who want to pursue this course are going to go forward and get the degree necessary and the skills necessary to become the managers and leaders we're going to need for tomorrow."

Blake Williamson, MD, MAM
Executive Director, Asante Health
Medford, Oregon

Blake Williamson was in a group practice in the Midwest back in the late 1980s when managed care growth was spurting in nearby Minneapolis. "We thought if we didn't do something like that, someone was going to come and do it to us. It was not a good reason to put up an HMO, but that's what we did. I think I was the only one who had any understanding of what the initials HMO meant, so I got appointed medical director," he recalls. "It didn't take me long to figure out that I wasn't comfortable, and I needed more training. Medicine is a lot clearer, as far as the type of decisions you make. In the business world, there's a lot more gray. I was uncomfortable with that grayness. That was a reason I went back to school."

Williamson was 38 years old and working with the Medical Arts Clinic in Minot, North Dakota, when he embarked on his MBA. His schedule was nightmarish; he says the only time he saw his children for two years was when they studied together. Still, he pursued the program and earned his Master of Administrative Medicine from the University of Wisconsin in 1990.

As he moved from medicine to management, Dr. Williamson did not realize how all-consuming management would become. In fact, he often reflected on how a physician executive's ideal job would include both clinical and leadership responsibilities. "I think the experience is more important than the degree," he says in retrospect. "The degree does help distinguish people, and I'd like to think it changed my perspective of the world. The physician is trained to look at the individual and at a single situation. In the business world, you get trained to look at populations and to try to manage the outcomes of them. That's changing a little, but not for the individual practicing physician."

Williamson already knew he could make a difference in a patient's life, but that was a short-term objective. He longed to produce a longer term effect and to trade the sameness of medicine for the challenge of administration. He believes he has got the opportunity to do just that at Southern Oregon Health Trust, which he joined last year as CEO. "The business world is a lot more frustrating at times, in that it takes a long time to get everybody rowing in the right direction," Williamson concludes.

J. Richard Gaintner, MD
CEO, Shands Hospital System, University of Florida
Gainesville, Florida

Richard Gaintner is no stranger to medical management. He's logged 29 years in the field and has been a CEO for the past 15. He says he's an alumni of the School of Hard Knocks, a veteran of the medical trenches who worked his way up the ranks over many years of hard work and courses through the American College of Physician Executives. "Ever since I was a little kid, I liked the idea of running things," he says with a laugh. "When I finally got into management, I wanted to run an organization and see if it was possible to do it in such a way that people enjoyed their work."

Gaintner was working at Johns Hopkins when he formally decided he wanted to be a CEO. "Being a CEO involves more leadership than management," he contends. "Particularly in a large organization where you can afford to have very talented people around you. Most important are interpersonal and listening skills, getting people to listen to you, to trust each other, and to realize that nobody has all the talent to do the job." But Gaintner points out that physician leaders not only have to have interpersonal skills; they must also be committed to taking care of communities.

Although he has no regrets about his journey to the top, Gaintner said he would definitely recommend that those aspiring to top management pursue a master's degree that's designed for physicians, such as the ones at the University of Wisconsin and at Tulane University. "My feeling is that there are still people like me and somewhat younger people who have come along without a degree. But, in the future, they'd be crazy not to get it," he says. "I'm relatively sure you can acquire knowledge without a degree, but I think, as more and more people get into management, the MBA will be the differentiation."

Gaintner predicts a rosy future for physician executives. "I'm very bullish on the future of physician executives," he says. "I don't think every doctor has the instincts to do it well and do it right, but, as physicians get advanced degrees, I think a lot of organizations will be looking for physician executives. It's important to get the word out."

Michael A. Stocker, MD, MPH
CEO, Empire Blue Cross/Blue Shield
New York, New York

Early in his medical career, Michael Stocker says he was idealistic and consumed with the concept of providing universal health care and outpatient medicine. With those thoughts in mind, he enrolled in the Master of Public Health program at the

University of Michigan in 1978. Unlike most of the physicians we interviewed for this chapter, Stocker is convinced that his success can be attributed solely to his track record for problem-solving, an art which often strays far beyond textbook cases. "I learned more from people who took the courses," he says. "Economics and finance were absolutely critical. Without courses in microeconomics and finances, I just don't think you can be a competent manager in the business. Most of the other things were interesting, but not necessary."

Stocker's first management position was at U.S. Healthcare (now Aetna U.S. Healthcare), where he says it was "incredibly difficult to convince them to put a physician in as manager." He believes there is a bias against physicians in large companies, particularly in senior management. "Usually they get hired when things really get screwed up; that's what creates the opportunity," he says. "If you're a medical director, which is how I started out, your place is assured. But once you try to step out of that role, you raise all kinds of negative reactions in the organization."

Stocker maintains that there are three ways to achieve the role of CEO: Bite the income bullet and get involved in an entrepreneurial start-up, work your way up in an organization, or take over a troubled organization. "CEOs have to come from someplace, so they're going to know a little more about one discipline than another," Stocker explains. "So, in the beginning—if they're smart—they spend a lot of time on things they don't know much about. And they learn quickly that they're never going to know enough to completely understand law or systems, for example, so the only thing they can do is to hire people who do those jobs well and hope. So, really, your ability to pick people is much more important than your knowledge of the area."

He further advises up-and-coming managers to take a pay cut and manage a clinic, then move up. "The way to get management positions is to say, 'I had this problem, and I solved it. Then, I had this bigger problem, and I solved that, too. And I did it by putting a team of people together.' Business is pretty much about what works," Stocker says. "If you want to be head of a company that has 100 shoe stores, you're much more likely to be president if you go run one of the stores than if you're an advisor to the current president."

Stocker firmly believes that "physicians can make a health care system work much more easily and much more efficiently and with much less capital than anyone else. The value of physician managers is that their experience may help them bring physicians together," he adds. "Physicians have very high authority needs and have a tendency to throw up weak leaders because they don't want to give up their authority to anybody. If physicians in general could learn to get along together and work cooperatively on things like outcomes data and cost data, they'd be much better off," he concludes. "My guess is that physician executives should be better at this than nonphysician leaders."

Conclusion

Some of these physicians worked their way up through the ranks over many years. Others shortened the trip to the top by obtaining an MBA or another advanced degree and accelerating the learning process. All agree that the strong interpersonal skills needed for the role of CEO cannot be acquired in the ivy halls, but there are technical and business skills that can be acquired in an advanced degree program or in a series of seminars similar to those offered by the American College of Physician Executives.

The consensus is that there is no substitute for on-the-job training and that physicians who want to get ahead should enhance that experience with committee leadership, networking, and mentoring, as well as by taking every opportunity to read and study more about medical management.

The road to the top is still not well traveled, but physician executives are blazing new trails every day. It is through these journeys that more and more physician executives will take their rightful place as leaders of health care. Only then will physicians truly be able to exert their influence on how health care is provided to their communities.

Chapter 17

The American College of Physician Executives

Howard J. Horwitz and Wesley Curry

The profession of medical management may be viewed as being born in 1975 with the founding of the American Academy of Medical Directors, now the American College of Physician Executives (ACPE, throughout this chapter the latter name will be used in all references to the organization). Physicians had been moving into responsible management positions, particularly in medical group practices and hospitals, prior to that time, but there is little evidence that either physicians or others viewed medical management as a profession until the emergence of ACPE. Health care management was a thriving profession, with most hospitals headed by nonphysician CEOs. Physician leadership roles still tended to be part-time and through election rather than appointment.

By 1975, however, the involvement of the federal government in health care delivery and financing through Medicare and Medicaid had altered the health care system irretrievably. Health care organizations were increasingly feeling a need to have physicians in leadership and management positions to oversee clinical functions. Physicians were being appointed to management positions, but their management skills ranged from slim to nonexistent. The presumption that physicians, because of their medical education and training, could easily adapt to the demands of management quickly proved false.

ACPE was founded by what is now called the American Group Practice Association to provide a professional home for this new type of medical practitioner and to provide educational programming that would better outfit these individuals for the rigors of management. The College's success over the years can be attributed to its single-minded attention to a two-prong objective—to assist physicians who might be interested in management to identify themselves and assess their qualifications for such roles and to then provide these individuals with all the tools they require for management success. Those objectives are achieved by a growing and changing array of career counseling, educational, informational, and advocacy programs.

Career Counseling

It is here that the path to medical management begins, or does not. The first decision is the most difficult, and the most momentous. Management is not for everyone. For those with the appropriate personalities and personal philosophies, management will prove an exhilarating and rewarding career choice. For those who fail to understand the nature of the shift from medicine to management, or who make the choice for "escape" rather than "achievement" reasons, the move can be short-lived and disastrous. The College's reason for involving itself in this decision-making process is obvious and at least partly self-serving—a bad decision does the physician no good, but it also does the medical management profession no long-term good to have excessive numbers of ill-suited management practitioners in its ranks. The College's "Career Choices" program offers the physician one way of testing his or her interest in management and of determining options once a positive decision is made. Both physician and spouse are encouraged to take the one-day course, which includes sessions on:

- **Life-Work Planning.** Discussions of why some activities energize and others drain, of how to incorporate energizing activities into professional and personal life, and of how best to prepare for career changes.

- **The Marketplace.** A discussion of the opportunities that are available in medical management, of the roles that physicians typically play in various types of organizations, and of the compensation those medical managers receive.

- **Job-Hunting Skills.** A discussion of the specifics of successful interviewing, of resume writing, and of networking for employment contacts.

Many of these career planning and management topics are also made available in one-on-one sessions at either College headquarters or at the physician's site. While all of this programming may be used to make basic career decisions, the content is also useful to physicians seeking to advance their careers or to improve their management effectiveness. All are aimed at helping actual and prospective medical managers to assess their strengths and weaknesses regarding management and to begin the process of acquiring and fine-tuning management skills.

Management Education Programming

Because the College and its leadership continue to believe that the educational route to management skills and competence should be as diverse as the membership of the organization, ACPE supports a wide range of educational opportunities and approaches. Its educational programming is predicated on the philosophy that continuing education is a fundamental building block for success. Professional growth is an ongoing and building process, and those who continue to grow will surpass those who fail to add to their knowledge base.

However, those who engage in continuing education must be sure that the activities they pursue are compatible with their personal and professional life-styles. Often, a negative outcome befalls the physician who takes on too much in too short a period. Opportunities for real understanding and growth are supplanted by an academic exercise. CME hours may accrue, but no real learning may take place, and with the misused time is lost opportunity to affect positive change for their patients and their organizations.

A New Way of Thinking

One of the greatest challenges facing clinical doctors as they enter the world of medical management lies not in the new content, but rather in their perceptions about the learning process. Throughout the physician's premed training and medical school course work, the emphasis has been on learning incontrovertible facts and then applying those absolute facts to a variety of case situations.

Management is not based on absolute facts. At best, it is based on a widely held collection of cause and effect relationships. Management is fraught with ambiguity and inconsistency. The rules of management are transitory and situation specific. Accurate interpretation and implementation of these managerial relationships are the hallmark of sound business management.

Physicians who pursue medical management must be prepared to re-learn the process of learning. Success in this new field will come to those who can comfortably operate in the shadows that lie between undisputed fact and best guess.

Physician in Management Seminars

The fundamentals of medical management are taught in the College's Physician in Management (PIM) series, three five-day courses taken in sequence to acquire exposure to general business and management principles and methodologies presented in a health care environment. The material in these courses starts at a basic level and builds as the modules are presented. Each seminar builds on its predecessor, and the previous seminar is the prerequisite for the next.

The sessions in the Physician in Management series are taught by separate faculty members who are experts in their fields. They are not medical practitioners with management experience. Each session is taught by a respected faculty member who brings years of real-world experience to his or her presentation. PIM faculty members come from industry, academia, and management consulting, and they are chosen not only for their command of the subject matter, but also for their ability to convey the information in a meaningful and informative fashion.

Physician in Management Seminar I. Starting with a global perspective on the health care industry, General Systems Theory attempts to explain how and why the industry behaves as it does. Health care economics and organizational finance give insight into the fiscal side of health care delivery. The health care marketplace is explored in light of positioning the organization to better meet the demands of all stakeholders, as is the evolving role of clinician into physician executive. Finally, in the last module, small group dynamics, meeting effectiveness, and problem-solving/decision-making skills are introduced.

Physician in Management Seminar II. Competition and conflict within organizational settings begins Seminar II. Modules on organizational power, communication effectiveness, and negotiating strategies and techniques are then presented. Building a strategic plan is one of the most critical segments of the second seminar. Ethical challenges of physician executives helps participants identify, prevent, and manage both managerial and clinical ethical conflicts within their organizations.

Physician in Management Seminar III. The last module of the series begins with an analysis of organizational change and the unique challenges it presents to medical leadership. Managing the quality of service addresses patient perceptions that go beyond quality of care indicators. A segment on creative problem solving is followed by the physician executive's role in managing organizational agreement and disagreement. Finally, the last module recaps the entire PIM series and offers advise on implementing the new skill set.

The College takes its own advice. Learning is a lifelong process. The Physician in Management series has evolved as the health care delivery system has changed. But the core content areas have remained fairly similar since the time these modules were first presented. It is the examples, cases, and texture that keeps adapting to the new structures and systems that define the industry. As the track record of these courses suggests, the content and the faculty have steadily provided the basic skill set to launch the beginning physician executive on the road to understanding and career advancement.

The Institutes on Health Care Leadership and Management

The Physician in Management seminar series provided the breadth; the College's Institutes provide the depth. Essentially on a quarterly basis, participants elect to explore a single medical management topic over the course of several days. The more intensive sessions are directed at the clinical doctor who has identified medical management as a career objective. Many times, management topics that are previewed in a one-day segment at the PIM are analyzed for two to four days at an Institute.

Among the topics presented at the Institutes are health law, medical information systems, managing physician performance, and financial decision making. Keeping pace with the changing marketplace, the College has recently launched a comprehensive curriculum in Management of Managed Health Care Organizations. Two, four-day programs explore managed care from the point of view of the staff model HMO and from that of the IPA or PPO health care provider. An additional one-day program introduces emerging issues in managed health care, giving participants early warning of changes that are just beginning to reveal themselves.

Among the topics presented at the Institutes are health law, medical information systems, managing physician performance, and financial decision making. Keeping pace with the changing marketplace, the College has recently launched a comprehensive curriculum in the Management of Managed Health Care Organizations and an Institute on Health Care Informatics.

The managed health care organization course is a comprehensive four-day program that focuses on the importance of value-based planning prior to implementing program or pricing structures, capitation of medical care, contracting issues, and the management of risk. The Institute on Health Care Informatics provides a changing menu of multiday courses that target trends in the utilization of information systems in medical settings. Among the topics at the institute are information systems for physician profiling, informatics of managed care, quality outcomes, and utilizing the internet for research and communication. There is also an introductory course on personal computing using Microsoft Windows.

As with the Physician in Management series, the core content of the Institutes remains somewhat constant from quarter to quarter. However, many of the sessions focus on emerging topics and must adapt to the changing environment to keep medical managers on the cutting edge of new trends and applications. The creation of the managed care courses is an indication that more in-depth courses were necessary to keep members abreast of the evolution of this delivery modality.

Advanced Standing and the Institute for Advanced Study

More seasoned health care executives may be granted advanced standing in the College. The pool for this honor is members and nonmembers who have achieved Certified, Diplomate, Fellow, or Distinguished Fellow status; who have earned an advanced management degree; or who have accumulated 150 or more credit hours in ACPE educational courses.

Those with advanced standing may be invited to attend College Institutes for Advanced Study, which provide focused, in-depth programs on critical medical management topics faced by the industry's top leaders. These courses emphasize problem solving, case analysis, and hands-on learning.

Courses offered at an Institute provide both the technical information and the context to further sharpen management and leadership skills. Each course is an in-depth exploration of a key management topic that goes beyond the introductory skills that are presented in other medical management courses. Therefore, acceptance into the Institute is limited to those who have already acquired a high level of educational and professional expertise.

To gain entry to a specific program in an Institute for Advanced Standing, the College member must be able to demonstrate special education or competence in the topical area of the program. This ensures that every participant has a solid foundation in the introductory concepts, thus allowing for a quick transition to the advanced issues in each managerial topic. The health care industry demands a distinctive set of managerial competencies. The Institute for Advanced Study was designed to build them.

Credentials in Medical Management

For many years, ACPE education courses, or their equivalent from other sources, were adequate for the demonstration of management skills. Those with the time and inclination could acquire advanced degrees, but on-the-job training and sound experience were probably the major source of differentiation among candidates in the recruitment for medical leadership positions.

However, in recent years, advanced educational credentials and additional certifications have become more widely desired by employers. This is particularly true in highly competitive situations, where work experience and a random selection of managerial courses is probably just not good enough. To help level a playing field occupied with senior physician executives, newer or younger physicians will want to be able to point to some credential that will help gain them acceptance.

Educational Credentials

ACPE has now developed an alternative to traditional graduate management programs that is based on its highly successful Certificate in Medical Management Program, now called the Graduate Program in Medical Management (GPMM). In GPMM, members of the College must complete a total of 218 contact hours in medical management education, containing a series of courses covering the depth and breadth of topics necessary for success in medical management. Each segment involves an examination that must be passed. The examinations may be taken at any ACPE educational program or electronically on the College's World Wide Web site.

Included in the required core is Physician in Management seminars I and II and courses on managing physician performance, medical quality management, management of change, health care finance, medical informatics, ethics, and health law. Electives may be selected from Physician in Management Seminar III, financial decision making, managed care, advanced informatics, interpersonal communications, and negotiation.

Following successful completion of the ACPE courses, GPMM enrollees must complete 72 contact hours in a Capstone Course at either Tulane University, New Orleans, Louisiana, or Carnegie-Mellon University, Pittsburgh, Pennsylvania. Upon sucessful completion, the College awards a Certificate in Medical Management. Those who possess the certificate may elect to continue the educational process by enrolling at Tulane University's Master of Medical Management Program. For those with the certificate, an additional three weeks of on-campus course work is all that is required to secure the degree.

Professional Designations

The "gold standard" in clinical medicine is board certification. Physician executives whose education and experience elevated them above their peers sought similar recognition. The American College of Physician Executives responded to this dilemma when it helped found the American Board of Medical Management (ABMM) in the late '80s. This organization, through a rigorous qualification and examination procedure, recognized with board certification physicians who demonstrated the required management competence. This board certification process may now be transferred to others within the American Board of Medical Specialties.

The Certified Physician Executive (CPE)

As the demand for physician executives has increased, required skills and competencies have increased as well. Success in medical management calls for preparation and education beyond that acquired during medical school and professional experience. Employers want medical managers to have credentials that go beyond their clinical designations. The Certified Physician Executive (CPE) designation recognizes demonstrated excellence as a physician executive.

The Certified Physician Executive designation is conferred on select physicians whose management education, demonstration of special competencies, and understanding of the field of medical management set them apart as having attained a superior level of management ability. The Certifying Commission in Medical Management (CCMM) grants the CPE designation.

The CPE designation is designed to ensure that physician executives:

- Have distinctive competencies and skills of value to organizations in the health care industry.

- Can effectively communicate those skills and competencies to a variety of constituencies.

- Have mastered the knowledge of medical management and can demonstrate managerial effectiveness.

- Can guide lesser experienced physicians in navigating the field of medical management.

Earning the CPE designation requires successful completion of a five-day skill-building tutorial and assessment presentation. The Tutorial provides a vehicle to better evaluate the ability to use and demonstrate the managerial skills required of today's physician leaders. To qualify for admission to the Tutorial a physician executive must:

- Be board certified in a clinical specialty recognized by the American Board of Medical Specialties.

- Provide a letter of recommendation from his or her immediate supervisor or a member of his or her organization's board.

- Have three years' clinical experience beyond residency training.

- Have one year's medical management experience.

- Complete the ACPE's Certificate in Medical Management Program, have an advanced degree whose curriculum is consistent with ACPE's certificate program curriculum, or complete 200 hours of management education that has been evaluated by examination and whose curriculum is consistent with ACPE's certificate program curriculum.

Advancement in ACPE

The CPE designation from CCMM may be the beginning of a route to formal recognition by ACPE of a physician executive's medical management credentials. The document from CCMM awarding CPE status may be used to apply to the College for Diplomate status. A College member who has achieved Diplomate status and has been a member for the past two years may apply for Fellow status, providing letters of nomination from two current Fellows or Distinguished Fellows of the College and from the CEO or governing body of his or her organization and evidence of contributions to the field of medical management. It is from the pool of College Fellows that the ACPE Board of Directors selects candidates for Distinguished Fellowship, the highest honor that a College member can achieve.

Advocacy

This expanding list of potential credentials in medical management, good as the College believes it is, will be of limited use if the organizations that hire physician executives are unaware of it or are unconvinced of the value of the credentials. Having put the credentials and the systems that support them in place, the College is now in the process of developing an advocacy program that explains the credentials and their value in hiring decisions, not only to physician executives, but also to hiring organizations and to recruitment firms that have substantial practices in the medical management arena.

An important element of this advocacy program will be forging close and mutually educational relationships with recruitment firms so that the medical management profession, how to succeed in it, and the value of ACPE credentials are better understood. This will make the College and recruitment firms partners in the placement of highly qualified physician executives.

The Role of Physician Executives in Selling the Profession

In the final analysis, it is physician executives themselves who will have the greatest impact on acceptance and growth of the profession. The array of credentials that can be obtained through the College will aid in their career advancement, particularly as the College intensifies its advocacy efforts. But the credentials are at best an entry ticket. In management, as in most professional endeavors, it is performance that makes the real difference. The ladder of credentials will be there to provide evidence of achievement, but it's achievement and honing of management skills that will distinguish physician executives. The duty of physician executives, to themselves obviously but also to the profession, is to be sure the skills are in place so that hiring organizations realize their value for their hiring decisions.

The College is committed to the development of educational programs and credentialing mechanisms that add to and document excellence in medical management, but management practitioners, as recipients of the results of these efforts, have the obligation of selling the value of the profession through proven performance and exemplary leadership.

Chapter 18

Reclaiming the Practice of Medicine: The Health Care Challenge of Our Age

by James J. Unland

Our health care system is at a dangerous crossroads.

The low road leads to a significant, irreversible increase in government regulation including the socialization or quasi-socialization of health care; the high road leads to opportunities for health care providers to reestablish a direct linkage of accountability and service with consumers in a way that will ensure the survival of a private, pluralistic health care delivery system in our nation. At no time has there been a greater need in the U.S. health care industry for physician executive leaders who understand the compelling need for health care providers to reclaim the practice of medicine and who are able to lead their colleagues in implementing highly evolved managed care in an enlightened, consumer-friendly manner.

The operative words here are "leaders," "enlightened," and "consumer-friendly."

Physician executives must be leaders able to educate their colleagues about managed care, aggregate their colleagues into physician networks, motivate their colleagues to participate in the vital reengineering of medical delivery, and forge alliances into regional networks with other health care providers (especially hospitals) to move up the "continuum of risk" and into direct contracting in its various forms.

Physician executives need to be enlightened, understanding that their power lies in the physician-patient relationship, the ability of physicians to advance the state-of-the-art in health care delivery, and the potential of physicians to ally with one another and with hospitals to form potent medical networks. Enlightenment also means recognizing that physicians can control their own destinies as long as they work together.

Finally (and above all else), physicians executives need to think in terms of creating and leading new kinds of consumer-friendly provider networks. The opportunity now lies before physicians and other providers to reclaim the practice of medicine by forming provider networks that create insurance products and services in their own right, establishing a direct linkage of accountability that can reverse recent trends by restoring consumers' confidence in a privately based health care system.

The frustration and anger of consumers cannot be overstated. Consumers are frightened that health care benefits are going to decrease, and they are gloomy about the future of our health care system, which many people describe as chaotic and increasingly impersonal. People repeatedly complain about hospitals with untrained caregivers, about too few real nurses staffing hospital floors, about physicians not answering questions adequately, about the underlying financial motivations of physicians, and about how difficult it can be to get a referral to a specialist.

Even more disturbing are comments to the effect that insurance companies are really controlling physicians and hospitals and that insurance and HMO middlemen really call the shots in the practice of medicine. But the most disturbing comments of all revolve around what many regard as the increasingly commercial and depersonalized nature of the health industry. Health care providers are regarded by many consumers as fixated more on profits than on caring for patients; physicians are viewed with suspicion by many people who wonder how physicians can put their patients first in the midst of all the financial incentives not to provide adequate care or, in some cases, not to even tell patients about all of their treatment options.

Many analysts, including a growing number of physicians, are questioning the fundamental direction our health care and insurance systems are taking. The insurance industry takes billions of dollars out of the health care system to act as middlemen. HMOs have large bureaucracies created to tell doctors how to practice medicine right down to the last detail; in many health plans, everything (even routine x-rays and drugs) requires "preauthorization" by a health plan administrator at the other end of an "800" number. Wall Street has gotten into the act, capitalizing mergers and acquisitions of health care entities and creating yet another diversion of funds away from direct patient care and toward return on investment.

Many people are asking some logical questions. Are all of these expensive middlemen really necessary? Why can not providers become directly accountable to consumers? Why can't provider networks self-regulate through committees of doctors with participation of hospital executives and consumers? If health care is to be rationed, should not consumers have some input into the process? Why do doctors need middlemen to tell them how to practice medicine; can not they get together by specialty and subspecialty and figure out how to practice in a high-quality yet efficient manner?

Managed care as we now know it is overly commercializing health care; creating built-in conflicts of interest for physicians; unnecessarily and dangerously interposing bureaucratic medical dicta on every facet of the practice of medicine; inserting more corporate middlemen and added costs; and, most unfortunately, eroding the relationship of trust between patients and physicians.

In the insurance industry's efforts to "manage" care, there seem to be some inherent conflicts of interest for physicians:

- Is a physician going to represent the best interests of the patient if any recommended treatment decision can ultimately affect that physician's compensation (either direct compensation or "bonus pool" participation)?

- Are primary care physicians going to attempt to take on too much patient care, going beyond their expertise in order to avoid referrals to specialists and possibly adversely affect their own bonuses?

- Will a physician recommend hospitalization if that is what is necessary, and, if so, will the patient be discharged prematurely?

- Will a physician inform the patient of the latest tests, procedures, and drugs if they are more expensive?

These and other potential conflicts of interest automatically assume greater proportions when physicians and hospitals—irrespective of the structural configuration of the contracting entity—begin to take on risk contracts with "withhold pools" and "bonus pools."

Potential conflicts of interest are even more pronounced when physicians work for nonprovider corporate management companies, often called PPMs (physician practice management companies). In such instances, physicians are working not only for themselves but also for stockholders of entities that are neither insurers nor providers; these entities are stock corporations that are "corporatizing" medicine by acquiring the assets of medical practices, entering into long-term contracts with physicians (often 20 years or more). One wonders who in his or her right mind would sign any management contract for 20 years.

These companies are management companies; they must still go out to contract with payers. Thus, the physician is driving a layered system of costs that must pay a desired rate of return to a Wall Street corporation and give payers themselves their "usual and customary" profit margins. With yet another layer of cost added to the insurers' 20-30 percent, physicians are pressured even more to ratchet down the amount and type of patient care to fit in the finite premium pool. Some of these corporations sweeten the deal for physicians by giving them stock or stock options. But whom does that help? With respect to these corporate "physician management" companies, the inevitable built-in underlying conflicts have become more pronounced—and potentially more serious from patients' point of view.

A growing number of people (including the AMA's own Council on Ethical and Judicial Affairs) believe that the fundamental relationship of trust between the physician and the patient is seriously compromised by all of these "incentive" programs and that patients will look skeptically at their physicians, wondering in whose interest they are really working. Patient mistrust of physicians could have another ripple effect, creating more demands for second opinions, more lawsuits, and higher administrative costs.

Fortunately, the number and percentage of physicians who have sold out to Wall Street management corporations is still quite small. In fact, many of the physicians who are approached by these companies and don't sell out cite, among other things, loss of independent clinical decision making as one of the reasons they decline such offers. Some have the attitude: "I'm already being driven crazy by insurance company UR people; now you want me to report to a bunch of Wall Streeters as well?"

Nonetheless, the consumer backlash against commercialized managed care is real, palpable, and dangerous. Consumer groups (aided by a liberal press all too delighted to publicize managed care war stories) have gotten the attention of many state and federal politicians. Anti-HMO "consumer protection" legislation has passed in one form or another in more than 40 states at this writing. Even more ominous, the Clinton Administration has set the stage for a major health care battle in 1998 by promulgating a consumer health care "bill of rights" in relation to consumers' knowledge about and interaction with health plans. Why is all of this government interference necessary? What brought this about? How far will it go?

The clear danger is that, if present trends continue, the consumer rebellion against commercialized managed care will, in a few years, drive us in the direction of some sort of nationalized health care system—in this author's opinion, a disastrous outcome. The challenge to all health care executives (especially physician executives) is to create provider networks whose paramount goal is restoration of trust between providers and consumers by making the linkage between these two groups as direct as possible.

Many providers are seriously considering new structures, organizations, and products designed to eliminate the middlemen, regain the practice of medicine, and establish a more direct relationship of accountability and service to consumers, providing health care efficiently while preserving patient choice and not compromising quality of care. Fortunately, at the same time that legislative bodies are considering additional "micro-management" of health care, some major legislative breakthroughs have occurred that open up significant "direct contracting" opportunities for provider networks, up to and including the formation of provider/insurer organizations.

Encouragement of Provider Networks from Governmental Entities

As most people in the health care industry now know, various states as well as the federal government have been working on one form or another of legislation and/or regulations that would permit health care providers to become insurers in their own right or at least be able to contract more directly with consumers by taking on "full-risk" contracts from HMOs and insurance companies while, commensurably, assuming additional "delegated authorities" with respect to such contracts with minimal interference from state insurance departments.

Although the various legislative and regulatory initiatives range widely, they tend to fall into three general categories:

- Initiatives that make it easier for provider networks to take on full-risk contracts with little or no insurance licensing and with less regulatory interference as long as those contracts run through legitimate existing insurance entities.

- Initiatives that permit provider networks to "direct contract" with self-insured employers and other self-insured organizations as long as such organizations meet certain definitions and insurance standards (in other words, as long as such organizations are truly "self-insured").

- Initiatives that would permit "direct contracting" between provider net works and consumers either on an outright basis or through some as yet unnamed type of insurance facility.

For the past few years, both Congress and many state governments have given various forms of "direct contracting" favorable attention. The initial ice was broken in Congress in 1995, when a far-sighted congressman from Illinois, Harris Fawell, introduced legislation that would permit provider networks to contract directly with self-insured employers without having to obtain state insurance licenses. (The legislation also would have permitted small companies and organizations to aggregate into self-insured entities). Not surprisingly, the National Association of Insurance Commissioners and all of the insurance lobbies vehemently and successfully opposed this legislation. (The legislation was not widely followed, and, at that particular time, most consumer groups and business trade associations stood on the sidelines). Nonetheless, the same concept was modified to apply to Medicare recipients—that is, provider networks would be able to direct contract with groups of the elderly subject to certain federal guidelines. This so-called provider-sponsored organization (PSO) legislation was introduced as part of the House Budget Resolution that passed in the House in November 1995 but did not pass in the Senate.

Since 1995, a number of bills that relate to both the commercially insured population and government programs have been introduced in this area. Recent activity has revolved around enabling provider networks to direct contract with Medicare or Medicaid recipients, subject to guidelines to be developed by HCFA, without the provider network itself having to obtain an insurance license in a given state. Other efforts in Congress relate to the commercially insured population, specifically enabling provider networks to direct contract with self-insured employers under the aegis of ERISA, again superseding state insurance departments.

Finally, in a groundbreaking move, Congress passed a new program with respect to Medicare to encourage provider networks to create their own "direct contracting" and PSO insurance capabilities. On August 5, 1997, President Clinton signed into law the Balanced Budget Act of 1997, following a summer of almost continuous negotiations between the White House and Congress.[1,2] In addition to addressing the federal budget itself, Section 4001 of the Act creates a new program under Medicare Part C, to be known as Medicare+Choice. Among other provisions, Section 4001 defines a PSO as "a public or private entity:

- That is established or organized and operated by a health care provider or group of "affiliated" health care providers.

- That provides a "substantial portion" of the health care items and services directly through the providers or affiliated group or providers.

- With respect to which affiliated providers share, directly or indirectly, substantial financial risk in the provision of such items and services and have at least a majority financial interest.

The law stipulates that health care "providers," as defined, may be any licensed provider, including physicians and hospitals. The law also provides that, in addition to the actual provider/owners of the PSO, other "affiliated" providers may be included in the PSO through contractual relationships.

The law calls on the Department of Health and Human Services (HHS) to devise guidelines that will govern certain aspects of the capitalization, licensing, organizational structure, and activities of PSOs. One feature of this Act that distinguishes it from the present environment is the ability of PSOs to apply for an explicit HHS waiver of state insurance licensing requirements if the PSO shows HHS that a state failed to act in a timely way on the required state insurance application or that a state has imposed solvency and other standards different from standards that HHS considers to be reasonable. In other words, PSOs do have to apply for state insurance licensure under this Act; however, if the PSO has difficulty with a state's insurance department and if the PSO meets certain solvency and other kinds of standards, the PSO could apply for and be granted a waiver from state insurance regulations, in which case federal standards and the federal waiver would supersede state laws.

The Act makes clear that HHS will develop further detailed guidelines during a rule-making process that has yet to occur as of this writing. Notwithstanding the fact that some details of implementation of this Act have yet to be worked out, the Act is unquestionably a significant and far-reaching development (some believe it the most dramatic development with respect to the Medicare program in decades). What would make this so? Several factors are noteworthy:

- PSOs could, in effect, become "insuring entities" under this legislation; thus, Medicare recipients would no longer need to go through approved "intermediaries" in order to participate in the program.

- Theoretically, many dollars can be freed up for providers and Medicare recipients alike.

- A more direct, more consumer-responsive linkage of service and accountability can be established between providers and consumers.

- The long-term solvency and viability of the Medicare program itself can be improved. This is, perhaps, the greatest underlying political reason why this legislation passed.

How will providers respond to this legislation? Across the United States, very few comprehensive, geographically regional provider networks even exist, let alone have the capability to become provider/insurers at this time. Still, this important legislation places heretofore unavailable opportunities at the feet of providers, and in many quarters it is thought that such opportunities will galvanize providers—especially hospitals and physicians—to put aside parochial, small-minded concerns and conflicts in order to make a determined effort to become better organized in their respective regions and to take steps to become Medicare provider/insurers in their own right.

Several questions arise. Do providers have the ability to really get together on a scale necessary to accomplish this? Can hospitals across regional areas really form effective contracting confederations that become PSOs? Can hospitals and physicians ever work together as partners in such an enormous venture, let alone amass critical numbers and coverage on a regional basis?

The answers to these and other related questions may only come with the passage of time. Even so, because of the enormity of certain "direct contracting" opportunities—and because of the absolutely essential role of physician executives within these contexts—it is instructive to more carefully examine the range of direct contracting configurations, the requirements of each, the characteristics of each, and some key elements for success. Before delving into the range of direct contracting activities available to providers, it is advisable to briefly describe what is meant by the "continuum of risk."

Defining the "Continuum of Risk"

Formation of insurance companies by providers is not the only option available to providers who recognize the goal of establishing a more direct linkage to the consumers they are supposed to serve. When the concept of taking on more risk by providers is discussed, it is important to understand that there is a "continuum of risk" that provides options other than simply setting up a provider-owned insurance company.

Levels on the continuum of risk can be characterized as follows:

Level 1: Contracting within Provider Category
This involves contracting with an independent insurance entity by taking on a risk contract that is applicable only to the specific type of provider entering into the contract. For example, a physician network would take on risk applicable only to physician services; a hospital network would take on risk applicable only to hospital services.

Level 2: A "Global" Risk Contract with an Outside Payer
In this type of contract, physicians and hospitals (and, possibly, other types of providers) would take "global" risk for a broad range of defined medical services, including home health care, rehabilitation, etc. Risk is taken either on a dollar premium basis or as a percentage of premium. The defining feature here is that the payer treats physicians and hospitals as a "unified provider." In these types of contracts, providers assume both financial risk and administrative functions; for example, utilization management and quality assurance are customarily "delegated" to providers under these types of contracts.

Level 3: A Joint Venture between Providers and an Insurer
Some joint ventures with insurance companies have been put together by provider networks. Although the specifics of these arrangements vary widely, they generally possess two common elements. First, the provider network and the insurer share joint ownership of an insurance entity, often a newly created entity. Second, utilization and quality management functions are most often totally delegated to the provider network, with the insurance company performing more traditional insurance functions, such as claims processing. Usually, both the insurer and the provider network contribute capital to such a venture.

It should be noted that "direct contracting" between a provider network and a self-insured employer would likely fall into this general position on the continuum of risk, because a self-insured employer would, for purposes of health insurance, be considered an "insurer" in its own right.

Level 4: Full Ownership of all Insurance Capabilities by Providers

Arrangements on this end of the spectrum can vary from outright acquisition of an existing insurance company or HMO by a provider network to start-up of a new insurance entity. Regardless of the specific configuration, providers own and control all services relating to both delivery of health care and insuring of health care.

Irrespective of the position of a provider network on the continuum of risk and irrespective of a provider network's other characteristics, two ingredients are essential to the assumption of risk in a profitable, successful manner:

● The provider network needs to have the financial capacity—either directly or through strategic alliances—to take on risk and reinsure in an appropriate manner.

● The provider network needs to be able to acquire and administer crucial functions relating to quality assurance, utilization management, "medical episode" management, and medical protocol development.

As provider networks move up the continuum of risk, the money they control increases, especially in relation to their ability to gain greater, or even total, control of insurance functions.

"Full-Risk" Contracting Between Provider Networks and Insurers[3]

Full-risk contracting occurs when providers take on master capitated contracts in one form or another from existing HMOs or insurers. There are several gradations of full-risk contracting and several types of configurations, depending on who is doing the contracting and the scope of the contract itself.

There are four general categories of full-risk contracting by provider type:

● Contracts that are "full-risk" for physician services only; usually the "master contract" is held by a physician group or network that is either strictly primary care or is dominated by primary care physicians.

● Contracts that are full-risk for hospital services only and that are held by hospitals themselves.

● Contracts in which hospitals and physicians jointly collaborate to hold a full-risk contract inclusive of both hospital and physician services.

● Contracts in which hospitals, physicians, and other providers, such as home health agencies, enter into a contract that is both full-risk and inclusive of all provider categories, thereby becoming truly "global" in nature.

Full-risk contracts may or may not come with "delegated authorities," which are specific functions that the insurer "delegates" to the provider network. Delegated authorities include activities such as physician credentialing, credentialing of other types of providers, utilization management, quality assurance, claims administration, and other similar functions. It is in the provider network's best interests to assume such functions, both because the provider network can be compensated for these activities and because the performance of these functions by a provider network has a higher likelihood of being conducted in a fairer, more consumer-friendly manner.

However, it is important to keep in mind that, from the payer's perspective, the payer remains accountable to policyholders under full-risk contracting, regardless of how many authorities are delegated to providers. Therefore, it is never in a payer's interest to simply saddle health care providers with a contract that they cannot administer. One arrangement that has been tried is the "administrative joint venture," in which providers take on a full-risk contract but rely greatly on the payer's management and infrastructure—at least for a time—to provide the tools for proper contract administration. Physicians and providers are still expected to execute "medical management" functions necessary to effect more efficient patient care delivery, but they do so using information tools and other organizational/management assistance from the payer with whom they are engaging in the full-risk contract.

Hence, in full-risk contracting arrangements, it is important to look not only at the assumption of medical and patient care risk by the provider network, but also the degree to which the provider network takes on truly delegated authorities.

The required effort and organization on the part of providers to administer full-risk contracts has been almost universally underestimated by the providers themselves. This seems to have been more true of physician-only networks than of physician-hospital networks or just hospital networks. Although little empirical information exists to explain these differences, one explanation is that hospitals and hospital systems had to develop sophisticated information systems and other infrastructure in order to cope with DRGs and other prospective payment systems in the 1980s. In addition, hospitals had to develop sophisticated financial information systems to support the multiple and challenging tasks involved in keeping track of information from a variety of payers throughout many hospital departments. Although hospital information systems still remain relatively unsophisticated when compared to the needs of highly evolved managed care, the fact that systems have been developed and are in place at many hospitals means that hospitals generally have more experience than physicians in managing information, reformatting information, etc.

Physicians, on the other hand, have operated by and large on a small scale, independently, and with unsophisticated infrastructure or none at all. Within the universe of medical practices, only a very small percentage of practices even today possess anywhere near the kinds of information systems and other management infrastructure to be able to undertake highly evolved managed care administration, and those that do tend to be larger group practices. The medical practice industry remains fragmented, notwithstanding publicity about some high-profile group practices and PPMs. These medical services organization (MSO) kinds of companies have not achieved much market penetration in relation to the total universe of physicians; moreover, many PPM companies that have acquired medical practice assets are often in a continued state of development of information systems and related infrastructure, delivering much less than is promised when the initial deals are made with the physicians themselves.

Therefore, although many types of providers are attempting to take on full-risk contracts, the ability to singularly and independently administer such contracts remains generally quite limited throughout the industry, both on the hospital and on the physician side, but especially on the physician side. Some collaborations between hospitals and physicians have produced more viable, more timely results in the areas of infrastructure and management; however, true collaborations of this kind are rare at present.

Regardless of who the contracting entity is, the following elements appear to be essential for a provider network to administer a full-risk contract:

- Ability to intelligently but fairly credential providers in a full-risk contracting network.

- In physician networks, ability to structure medical management/quality assurance committees by specialty, with committees meeting regularly to review existing utilization patterns and develop treatment protocols.

- In hospital networks, ability to assemble physicians and key hospital personnel to be able to regulate utilization across the network and within the hospital and to develop or adopt "critical paths" by DRG or by encounter type.

- Development and implementation of an information systems infrastructure that can "uplink" patient encounter data from the operating unit level (whether it be a medical practice, a hospital, a home health agency, or all of the above) and reaggregate that information into intelligent medical management tools that permit utilization and quality management within the network as well as development of treatment protocols and critical pathways.

- In physician-hospital networks that are collaborating on a full-risk managed care contract, understanding and acceptance of goals that are developed as well as of specific financial arrangements that provide mutual as well as respective motivations on the part of all parties to successfully execute and administer the contract.

- Full disclosure by payers of all demographic and medical characteristics of the population being insured under the full-risk arrangement, and cooperation by payers with the provider network so that risk parameters can be identified.

- An adequate cost accounting and cost finding structure within the provider network, especially relating to more costly items, such as specialists procedures, diagnostic tests, and any kind of hospital encounter.

Weakness in or inattention to any of the above areas can seriously hamper the provider network with respect to effective contract administration. If information tools are not present, for example, physicians are not going to be able to police their colleagues, much less engage in any sophisticated managed care behavior, such as development of treatment protocols. Even having advanced information tools available is no guarantee of effective risk contract management; an unfortunate fact of life in many provider networks is that one of the more challenging tasks is to persuade physicians to attend meetings, analyze data, and literally change the way they think about practicing medicine.

Hospital-physician relations can be a significant barrier to the development of managed care infrastructure capabilities with respect to full-risk contracting. For example, if goals and rewards are not mutually and respectively accepted by both physicians and hospital executives, attempting to practice efficient medical management will inevitably create conflicting loyalties, arguments about what "effective" medical management really means, and incessant quarreling about referral patterns, hospital outpatient utilization, and other issues where control of money always lies just beneath the surface.

In full-risk arrangements with physicians, hospitals must always place themselves in a position in which their goals are such that the hospital executives can genuinely feel free to encourage physicians to direct and engage in policing, medical management, and protocol development activities that fundamentally change the state-of-the-art of the practice of medicine itself and the delivery of patient care on a systemwide basis, thereby living up to the potential of successful full-risk contracting. Otherwise, the underlying motivation on the part of all parties to engage in highly evolved managed care will never be present, causing opportunities in full-risk contracting to be limited and the potential of such contracting never to be reached. Therefore, effective contract administration requires not only technical support and infrastructure tools but also the motivation and will power to engage in such activities.

It is vital that any provider network—whether physician-driven, hospital-driven, or some other configuration—recognize that negotiating the medical risk aspects of a full-risk contract is not the only negotiation that takes place. Negotiating the specific types of "delegated authorities" and the financial implications and arrangements with respect to such authorities are important elements of full-risk contracting discussions. Because it is not uncommon for insurers to charge in the range of 25 percent of every premium dollar for underwriting medical risk and for what they call "contract administration and profit," providers and provider networks should recognize that it is always in their best interests to take on as many delegated authorities as they can competently administer and, simultaneously, be compensated for doing so.

Some provider networks—wisely—have taken the philosophy that contract administration activities should be undertaken strictly on a break-even basis. The philosophy here continues with the notion that providers should be making bonuses and net profits with the intelligent management of patient care and the efficient delivery of health care services and that insurance functions inclusive of utilization and quality management should be undertaken as a management support service that does not make money and is not "marked up." This approach presupposes that a provider network is fundamentally better positioned to engage in medical management and other sophisticated managed care administrative functions than an insurer, as long as the provider network is properly organized and is supported by the proper infrastructure. Theoretically, then, functions that are taken over by the provider network from the insurer and that are no longer marked up by the provider network can be accomplished more efficiently and, in the end, actually free up dollars that can be put into more patient services, more provider bonus pools, lower premiums, or a combination of all of these.

Unfortunately, very few provider networks have reached a scale and degree of sophistication to be able to take on delegated authorities in such a way as to free up net dollars. It is this author's strong belief, however, that this will happen as provider networks become larger, thereby creating more economies of scale; as these networks become more organizationally sophisticated in their ability to assemble and motivate physicians and other medical talent to undertake advanced "medical management"; and as competition from the aggressive "direct contracting" kinds of networks forces a restructuring of both the concept and the implementation of full-risk contracting itself.

The two most prevalent forms of full-risk contracting are physician-only full-risk contracts and hospital-physician full-risk contracts under the aegis of physician-hospital organizations (PHOs). Physician-only full-risk contracts tend to cover only physician services and not hospital services. Many of these contracts are undertaken between insurers and primary care physicians, who hold the "master" contract and whose responsibility it is to administer all physician services under that contract, including specialty services.

Multispecialty physician group practices and IPAs have also engaged in full-risk physician contracts that, most commonly, leave hospitals out of the contract. Once again, the idea of these contracts is to draw a circle around all physician services and allow physicians to administer those services on behalf of insured populations. Although some of these contracts have been quite successfully administered, many have not. Several problems have occurred with respect to physician full-risk contracting:

- Some small and medium-sized primary care physician groups have taken on full-risk contracts for defined populations without understanding what is involved in medical management.

- Primary care physicians too often continue their old practice patterns and old referral patterns, not realizing that referrals to specialists and, in some cases, to hospitals can greatly affect financial performance under the contract.

- Many medical practices taking on full-risk contracts simply do not have the infrastructure and information tools to administer the contracts.

- Many IPAs and physician networks taking on full-risk contracts, likewise, do not have the infrastructure tools or do not know how to use the tools they have; in some cases, management tools were simply not available and in other cases were available and were not utilized. This could be the fault of physicians themselves, the fault of management of an IPA (or group practice), or a combination of both.

- Physicians may not have been alert enough or sophisticated enough to negotiate a proper capitated rate in the first place. Payers cannot always be blamed for poor rate setting in rate negotiations. Even though payers are, of course, trying to be as competitive as possible in their respective market, it does not make sense for a payer to negotiate a full-risk capitated rate with physicians in which the physicians are destined to fail from day one, because the ultimate liability for medical loss excesses often falls back on payers, especially if the IPA or group practice becomes insolvent.

Full-risk contracting by physicians most often fails because the physicians do not know what they are getting into, do not realize the extent to which they need to change their practice behavior, do not have the tools to undertake advanced medical management, and do not have or are unwilling to invest the capital to put sophisticated information systems and other infrastructure in place. This is not to say that full-risk contracting on the part of physicians is always a failure. Some larger group practices have quite successfully engaged in full-risk contracting, and a few have gone even to the point of "global" contracting, in which they take on not only physician medical risk but hospital and ancillary risk. (More commonly, however, full-risk contracting by such groups is restricted to physician-only risk).

Some smaller medical groups have been able to take on full-risk contracting successfully when an insurance company, HMO, or hospital (in a PHO type of structure) helps the group with administrative support or enters into some sort of administrative joint venture with the group. This kind of outside support has been provided to IPAs in some instances where full-risk physician contracting has been successful. At the same time, very few IPAs or POs have been able to enter into full-risk contracting without either raising significant capital among their members (which is rare) or taking in some kind of partner.

The most common partners with physicians entering into full-risk contracting are, of course, hospitals. Generally speaking, hospitals and physicians have always been viewed as logical contracting partners for the following reasons:

- The provision of most health care services—particularly acute care services and routine medical services—is carried out by and large between hospitals and physicians over a "continuum" of care (it should be acknowledged that the home care industry can be regarded as a recent and important player in highly evolved managed care).

- Most hospitals have capital and are willing to invest capital for important elements such as information systems, management, and other managed care "infrastructure." The vast majority of physicians are unwilling to invest the amounts of capital needed for the establishment of full-risk contracting capabilities, although there are a few notable exceptions.

- In any highly evolved managed care effort, hospitals and physicians really do need to work together to "reengineer" the practice of medicine. It is not enough for physicians to change their referral patterns and develop their own treatment protocols, because the hospital component of cost is very high in many medical episodes. Therefore, paying attention to the hospital component of staffing, supplies, workflow, and other matters can be an important element in reducing costs, and one of the most common ways of accomplishing this is for physicians and hospital staff to collaborate in the development of "critical paths."

- There are often significant administrative and marketing cost savings that motivate hospitals and physicians to collaborate on a managed care contract. This is especially true if the contract contains "delegated authorities" for the hospitals and physicians.

- Increasingly, payers are interested in full-risk contracting with as few provider entities as possible, as long as those entities are able to administer their end of the contract and the provider network covers a large enough geographic and population catchment area to make the overall effort worthwhile.

The most common vehicle for full-risk contracting by hospitals and physicians in collaboration with one another has been the PHO. Although at one time PHOs were widely regarded as the answer to providers' challenges with managed care contracting, they have been found to have a number of limitations:

- Many single-hospital PHOs have been too limited in geographic and population coverage.

- Single-hospital PHOs often do not have the capital to invest in complex systems and administrative support.

- Many PHOs do not have enough medical staff members to make them worthwhile.

- Many PHOs have been criticized by physicians for "stacking the deck" in favor of hospitals from the point of view of control of governance, contracting, rate-setting, allocation of receipts, and bonus pools.

- Some PHOs have jumped into risk-contracting without really understanding the full process and without obtaining the necessary time commitments on the part of a large enough number of physicians to be able to effectively assume delegated authorities and undertake other medical management efforts.

One approach to hospital-physician collaboration that seems to be supplanting the more traditional PHO approach in many markets is a partnership or joint venture between a hospital/hospital system and an independent IPA or PO. There have been numerous instances in which established IPAs were able to get together with hospitals or hospital systems and work out a joint full-risk contracting approach. These instances often involve far different revenue sharing and management arrangements than traditional PHOs. Some positive features of these kinds of arrangements are as follows:

- When an independent, established IPA or PO is coming to the table to discuss joint contracting efforts with a hospital, it is likely that the physicians have already accomplished at least some basic degree of organization among themselves. This is contrasted with many PHOs, which start out by attempting to bring together widely disparate individual members of their hospitals' medical staffs who have never collaborated in any fashion.

- Some IPAs and POs are established enough in their own right to have management and at least some infrastructure in place and have had experience with managed care contracting, including full-risk capitated contracting with respect to physician services. Even if this management staff and this contracting experience are regarded as rather basic, the established physician organization brings to the table a great deal more than is the case with most PHOs, which may just be starting out with an effort to organize independent physicians.

- Existing IPAs and POs that have already engaged in some medical management experience have the advantages of understanding what medical management is all about prior to getting involved with hospitals. Furthermore, conducting credentialing, utilization management, quality assurance, and other efforts such as treatment protocol development forces physicians in an IPA or a PO to work together, attend meetings, and focus on the important points at hand. This kind of experience can be an enormous advantage for hospitals attempting to collaborate with physicians, because the physicians already understand the basics of managed care and risk management.

Many hospitals have tended to view independent physician organizations as a threat rather than as a potential ally. In the past two or three years, however, this thinking has changed among most enlightened hospital executives. For one thing, attempts to organize medical staffs into PHO structures have often been frustrating. Second, it is well known among physicians and hospital executives that the medical community views PHOs with a great deal of skepticism. Third, the attainment of large physician numbers in a contracting federation with a hospital or hospital system is often much easier through an IPA structure than through a PHO structure.

Physicians often feel that it is important for them to be able to negotiate with hospitals on a partnership or "parity" basis and that this is much better done through an organization that they own and control as an independent entity that can come to the table to meet hospitals on a more equal basis than might otherwise be the case. A number of hospitals and hospital systems have dramatically revised their thinking in this entire area and have taken proactive steps to approach existing IPAs and POs with the goal of establishing a contracting federation. In some instances, the respective organizations establish a limited liability corporation that has as its "members" a hospital system and an IPA. In other instances, hospitals and IPAs have established a PHO through some type of merger in which hospitals and physicians own the PHO in equal portions but in which physicians have a great deal more control than they might have had in more traditional, older types of PHO structures.

The ultimate struggle for ownership and control of managed care contracting between hospitals and physicians is, of course, linked to money. Money flows in two ways to providers under most full-risk master contacts. First, there is usually a division of the total capitated rate among "physician services" and "hospital services." In addition, there is the creation of a "bonus pool" or "incentive pool" that may take on several different forms and have several different components.

The struggle over control of the allocation of money can be enormously complicated in hospital/physician contracting federations. Just the definition of what medical services are categorized as "physician" services versus "hospital" services can be a major bone of contention, especially as it relates to outpatient and ambulatory services, where a hospital is providing medical care that can also be obtained in a physician's office. When physicians or IPAs own surgical centers and diagnostic centers, allocation of capitated dollars in these activities can also become a difficult negotiating item.

The issue of relative capital contributions can be decisive. Physicians often want a hospital to pay for just about everything in the belief that physicians are bringing value to the table by virtue of an organized IPA or PO. Leaving aside the fact that this can bring up a whole series of legal/regulatory issues, hospitals often insist that physicians make at least some investment in the venture in cash. Likewise, when funds are going to be borrowed from an outside source to capitalize the venture, hospitals generally like to see physicians or the physician entity "on the hook"—at least to some extent—with the hospitals.

Most contentious of all can be the allocation of bonus pool monies. On the one hand, physicians realize that the largest single source of bonus pool money comes from reduced hospital utilization, especially reduced inpatient utilization. Because they are making the decisions about whether or not to hospitalize patients, physicians often feel that the majority of savings with respect to the so-called "hospital incentive pool" should go to them. On the other hand, hospital executives assert that, even though hospital utilization may decline under a full-risk capitated contract, the hospital still needs to maintain a competent staff and keep facilities up to date. In addition, the hospital may incur expenses for infrastructure, marketing, administration, and other activities related to the contracting venture and may feel a legitimate need for a return on these investments, all of which benefit the physicians as well as the hospital.

It is beyond the scope of this chapter to suggest compromises that might be explored among the parties when hospitals and physicians attempt to collaborate in a master full-risk contract. What can be said here is that there is no substitute for a full understanding on the part of all parties of the implications of what it means to be a "partner." True partners understand what each party brings to the table. They understand the respective strengths and weaknesses of each party and the added value of each. True partners also understand what it means to take financial risk in a business venture, and there is no question that a full-risk managed care contract is a business venture. In the health care industry, partners who happen to be health care providers also need to understand that payers and consumers do not really care who controls bonus pools or even how the capitated dollar is divided among providers. What the payers and consumers want from providers are responsiveness, value, and comprehensiveness of services.

Full-risk managed care contracting between health care providers and insurers is also beginning to involve other players, such as home health agencies. Even though at this time hospitals and physicians are the major parties to such contracts, other types of providers, such as home health agencies, rehabilitation companies, and mental health professionals, are going to want to come to the table. In fact, hospitals and physicians will want these other parties at the table, especially if they begin to take full-risk "global" health insurance contracts from payers that cover the full range of medical episodes. Whereas, in the past, home health care, rehabilitation medicine, and psychological counseling might have been considered "fringe" services, these and other services can be vital to successful administration of a full-risk contract that purports to provide comprehensive health care to a defined population.

Therefore, three major forces are expected to be at work with respect to full-risk contracting:

- Such contracts will become increasingly "global" in nature, encompassing the full array of health care delivery.

- As a result, the types of health care providers that become parties to such contracts and are included in provider networks will expand.

- Provider networks will, increasingly, acquire the capability and the confidence to assume more "delegated authorities," and they will take on additional contract administration responsibilities, for which they will be compensated by the insurance companies by virtue of receiving a greater percentage of the premium dollar.

Joint Ventures between Providers and Established Insurers

In recent years, some provider networks have entered into a variety of types of arrangements with existing insurance companies and/or HMOs that involve more than an arm's length full-risk contracting relationship. A few of these new kinds of arrangements will be described here, but before doing so it is important to point out the motivations on each side that lead to what can loosely be described as "joint venture" arrangements between providers and insurers.

- Provider networks may see opportunities in a specific market to develop a "proprietary"—or what is often called a "private label"—insurance product. This is in line with efforts to be more directly responsive to consumers. In addition, a provider network that establishes a private label insurance product is also able to market both the network and the insurance product, thereby cultivating a singular image in the market. Most sophisticated provider networks realize that, although name recognition and a reputation for quality are important in their marketing efforts, consumers are making decisions about insurance products based on features over which the providers often have little control. Fundamentally, the private label concept is part of an effort to increase market share and enhance image simultaneously.

- Money is, of course, a major motivation in any business venture. Provider networks that joint venture with existing insurers are most likely in a position to take more financial risk than they otherwise would even in a full-risk contract, but the rewards also can be significantly greater. From the point of view of providers, if they are confident that they can undertake highly evolved medical management while, at the same time, be successful in marketing an insurance product and preserve a reputation for high-quality patient care with comprehensive services, the provider network can do well financially, depending on the specifics of the joint venture arrangement with the insurer.

- Some providers believe that they need to be a partner with an insurer in order to obtain the information and the medical management tools necessary to undertake highly evolved managed care. A partnership or a joint venture arrangement most often motivates all the parties to share information, because they are now working toward a common goal as partners rather than having separate goals as providers contracting with insurers. This "mutuality of goals" in a provider-insurer partnership arrangement can eliminate duplication of certain efforts while, at the same time, bring ing expanded and more sophisticated capabilities to the venture.

- From an insurer's perspective, having a provider network as a partner causes providers to be more motivated to participate in highly evolved managed care activities, even more so than might be the case with just a full-risk contract. This is especially true if the joint venture is a partner ship in which the parties are at risk with capital, joint marketing efforts, etc.

- Some insurers believe that their liability exposure in managed care situa- tions is going to significantly increase in the coming years. "Liability expo- sure" used in this context means exposure to lawsuits as a result of claims denials, strict utilization patterns, denials of physician or other provider membership in a network or on a panel, etc. In addition, it appears that there is a growing anti-HMO consumer movement, as evidenced by the recent California ballot initiative and other legislation throughout various states. The thinking on the part of some insurers is that, by having providers in partnership with more of a team concept, providers will be partially responsible for making the tough decisions regarding the alloca- tion of resources and the combined organizations will be able to market in a way that results in a more positive public image.

It is important to be able to distinguish between true joint venture arrangements and full-risk contracting arrangements. Some of the features that are necessary in order for a collaboration between providers and an insurer to qualify as a true joint venture are as follows:

- The provision of medical services needs to be comprehensive, at least as comprehensive as the schedule of benefits normally marketed by the insur- er. In other words, in a provider/insurer joint venture arrangement, con- sumers should receive at least the same benefits that they would have received from the insurer solely and directly. In order to market itself more effectively and to create a positive, differentiated image among consumers, it is advisable for provider/insurer joint ventures to attempt to expand the benefits schedule as much as possible.

- There should be true joint ownership of either an independent entity or, at least, a specific array of products. It is nearly always advisable in a provider/insurer joint venture for the parties to create a new, separate legal entity that they co-own on some basis and through which all activi- ties and funds are channeled, including specially "branded" products. The alternative to creation of a separate legal entity is creation of a product that is particular to the joint venture. In this approach, the insurance com- pany and providers create a product that is, technically, developed under the aegis of the insurance company but that is actually developed and mar- keted by both the insurance company and providers and in which the providers share substantial ownership as well as financial risk and reward.

- A true joint venture possesses legitimate financial risk sharing by both providers and the insurer. One of the distinguishing differences between this approach and a simple "full-risk" contract is that risk sharing in a joint venture is total, meaning that financial risk for medical services is shared over the entire array of products and services and that at least some financial risk for product development, marketing, administration and reinsurance is borne by providers.

- Information systems and administration are unified under one team. In a joint venture, there is no longer any incentive for an insurance company to withhold special information from providers; there is every incentive for the insurer to want the providers to be as successful as possible and to have as much highly formatted information as possible to undertake sophisticated medical management. Likewise, a true joint venture central izes functions such as credentialing, quality management, treatment protocol development, marketing, and claims administration under a team concept, recognizing that the configuration of committees and task forces will be weighted variously by committee, depending on the function to be performed. For example, the parties may agree that the insurer will handle claims administration and that the task force responsible for that activity will contain only one or two representatives from the provider network. On the other hand, medical management and quality assurance may be weighted very much in favor of provider representatives on those task forces. The delineation of committee and task force composition is normally structured on a logical, functional basis in which functions more naturally handled by providers tend to be associated with committees that have greater provider representation, while those functions more naturally handled by the insurer tend to be handled by committees more dominated by insurer representatives.

- The true joint venture seeks to market a health insurance product or array of products as a combined entity and in such a way as to differentiate the joint venture's products from all others in the market. Hence, in this kind of joint venture both providers and the insurer are each conducting marketing efforts in a "push-pull" fashion that can, if undertaken properly, be extremely effective.

In any type of provider/insurer joint venture—regardless of the specifics of ownership and control—the goal of product differentiation in the marketplace cannot be overemphasized. It makes no sense from either providers' or insurers' points of view to go to the trouble of creating a joint venture in the first place unless there are some market positioning advantages of doing so. If providers are just looking for a greater share of responsibility in a managed care contract, they might as well stick to a full-risk contract that has delegated responsibilities with the accompanying compensation. Likewise, if an insurer is simply looking to transfer more responsibilities to providers and motivate providers to undertake more advanced medical management etc., this can be accomplished through a full-risk contract in conjunction with delegated authorities.

It is the potential to accomplish something more ambitious in a given market that should be the fundamental motivating factor as well as the overriding objective in any provider/insurer joint venture. The mere existence of a joint venture is not in itself reason to undertake such a project. Consumers really do not care about new kinds of health care organizational schemes; they respond to differentiated products and services. Thus, any contemplated joint venture between providers and insurers in a given market should be undertaken only with some important market-based objectives in mind:

- An attempt should be made to create more comprehensive health care insurance products and services for consumers than are available from traditional insurers. Within each product area, the joint venture should attempt to structure additional services for consumers that, once again, differentiate the joint venture from all other insurance products in the market. The very last image that such a joint venture wants to portray is of "just another insurance company" in the market.

- Several different programs should be offered, giving consumers a choice of programs with corresponding pricing variations.

- The provider network should have as wide a membership of providers as possible, especially physicians and hospitals and including "contracted" providers.

- The provider network should cover as much of a geographic population catchment area as possible, and the "defined" market should be geographically delineated to include a logical market definition area based on people's living and working patterns. This is particularly true if the provider network and the insurer are going to cover commercial lives through the joint venture.

- Choice of physician by consumers should be a backdrop of all product development efforts.

- The name and other "branding" features of the joint venture and its specific insurance products should be distinguished from the name of the insurance company. In some cases, a name associated with a provider network could be beneficial, depending on specific circumstances.

- Emphasis should be placed on community service and the benefit to consumers of this joint venture. Wherever possible, consumers should share in the savings from highly evolved medical management and should be motivated to undertake preventive health care. In addition, some of the system savings freed up by improved management and lower utilization should be passed along to consumers in either premium reductions or expanded benefits. Every effort should be made to avoid the image of the joint venture as some kind of "sweetheart deal" between providers and an insurance company that is going to benefit only those parties.

The creation of a proper market image in a joint venture of this kind—backed up and underpinned by solid, consumer-friendly products—is the most important characteristic that will distinguish such an effort in the market and permit both providers and the insurer to accomplish greater market penetration than would be the case with just a full-risk contract or some other more traditional managed care arrangement. Because perception and image are so vitally important in the health care industry today—especially in light of all the anti-HMO publicity of the past two or three years—it is advisable for a provider/insurer joint venture to have actual consumer representation on the board of the entity being created and even on key committees. It is beyond the scope of this discussion to suggest these kinds of steps in more detail except to say that listening to the concerns of consumers and structuring products and organizations accordingly is both common sense and good business policy.

A provider/insurer joint venture in which the hospital provider component contains not-for-profit community hospitals possesses some potential advantages over other types of configurations. First, most not-for-profit hospitals have a history of community service. Second, not-for-profit hospitals do not have to make a profit on the insurance functions of a provider/insurer joint venture, although, of course, they still need to be involved in a venture that attains a positive cash flow. Because not-for-profit hospital networks do not have pressure to generate a return on investment to Wall Street, they can focus on the mission at hand, which is to provide health care services that contain value and have appeal to consumers.

Dealing with the physician component of a provider/insurer joint venture arrangement can be quite challenging and should not be underestimated. Hospitals and insurance companies need to recognize and accept up front that it will simply not be possible to structure a differentiated array of health care insurance products at competitive prices without active and enthusiastic involvement of physicians. Ultimately, it is physicians who must do the day-to-day work to improve the state of the art of medical management, and it is this advanced medical management that, in turn, creates efficiencies in the system. Although efficient hospitals and good home health agencies can also greatly contribute to systemwide efficiencies, "medical management" really means changing the way medicine is practiced by physicians, because physicians make nearly all of the decisions governing resource allocation and utilization.

Several general points can be made with respect to physician involvement in a provider/insurer joint venture:

- Involving physicians at the earliest stages of conceptualization is most helpful. Any project in which the initial impetus comes from hospitals will automatically be viewed with suspicion by a great majority of physicians because of historic tensions that most rank-and-file physicians and hospitals have experienced over the years. Wherever possible, hospitals and hospital systems should avoid getting ahead of physicians with respect to provider/insurer joint venture discussions, or physicians will always feel they are playing to a "stacked deck" in which hospitals and the insurance company are planning to take advantage of them.

- Physicians and hospitals that enter into discussions regarding a joint venture and that bring prior experience with full-risk contracts have a significant advantage over providers without full-risk contracting experience. In fact, prior experience with full-risk contracting on the part of providers is almost an essential precondition to entering serious discussions about a true joint venture with an insurance company. Although it is theoretically possible to embark on a joint venture without prior full-risk contracting experience, numerous aspects of the project become more difficult and time-consuming without such experience. As stated previously, parties who have had such experience have often been able to work out their political and financial differences, and they share a history of functioning together in a collaboration to improve the state of the art of medical management.

- Collaboration between an IPA and a hospital in joint contracting can become the basis for the provider side of a joint venture agreement with an insurance company. Once again, if the IPA (or the PO) and the hospital or hospital network are already engaged in successful risk contracts, with committee structures and administrative capabilities already in place, this is a significant advantage in joint venture projects with insurance companies. Even more fundamentally, in situations in which physician networks and hospitals have experience working together, physicians not only are less likely to view the joint venture concept with suspicion but are also more likely to embrace the concept and see its market potential and business potential for them.

In approaching a provider/insurer joint venture of any kind, one needs to be starkly realistic about the attitudes of physicians, or the project will fail. Physicians are not charities and do not operate their businesses as such. Physicians do care about their patients, but they view any project in the managed care arena—especially ventures with hospitals or insurers—with a question: What's in it for me? Most community-based physicians are in business to make money practicing medicine, and the view of many physicians around the country is that managed care and government efforts are conspiring to limit or reduce their incomes.

On the other hand, more enlightened physicians understand what managed care is all about and are receptive to going to the trouble to change the way medicine is practiced, as long as there is something in it for them—more patients; a more secure market position; and, above all, greater compensation. For example, if physicians go to the trouble to attend meetings and agonize over medical protocols, utilization standards, and quality assurance and if all of these efforts create managed care bonus pools of one sort or another, the physicians want at least an equal share of such bonus pools. Anyone who has ever been involved in negotiating full-risk contracting arrangements with respect to the distribution of income between physicians and hospitals understands that a large number of issues can create stress and conflict, not just in the initial negotiations but also in ongoing administration of the contract.

Hence, when physicians approach a joint venture among providers and an insurance company, many of them wonder why they should get into any kind of partnership arrangement with entities that many regard as historic adversaries and how they can ever be treated fairly in such an arrangement, notwithstanding what the other parties may say about the potential of the joint venture. As mentioned previously, the single best way to mitigate such perceptions on the part of physicians is a past and ongoing relationship in full-risk contracting in which physicians have already worked out some kind of acceptable ownership and governance structure with the hospital and have already experienced financial rewards by virtue of participation in a bonus pool over and above what they would otherwise have received in the routine practice of medicine.

Some joint venture concepts envision giving physicians majority ownership control of the provider side of the equation. Others envision the creation of a for-profit MSO that becomes the administrative arm of the joint venture and in which the physicians own a significant amount of stock. Physicians love to own stock in medical organizations, and they are often enthralled by the notion that, at some time in the future, this stock could be worth a great deal of money. This is the approach that Wall Street MSO companies use to entice physicians into their fold.

Although some of these ideas may be good ideas in particular circumstances, there is one overriding financial motivation for physicians that, if structured properly, should cause them to consider the provider/insurer joint venture concept more seriously then they would other kinds of arrangements. A provider/insurer joint venture has the potential for physicians to make a great deal of money simply practicing medicine in the right way. Physicians need to be shown that they can participate in significant financial benefits if medical management is conducted properly, given a population that is paying in constant premium dollars.

In structuring joint venture arrangements, both the hospital parties and the insurance parties to the arrangement need to recognize that it is the "here and now" financial potential of good medical management that will encourage physicians to think differently about the joint venture's potential than they do about PHOs, risk contracts, and other structures. In addition, the fact that a joint venture is really an arrangement among partners, with the potential to participate in total premium dollars—not just premium dollars after the insurance company has skimmed off its portion—differentiates joint ventures from other contracting arrangements.

No joint venture among providers and an insurer can succeed without the involvement of large numbers of physicians in a geographic/population catchment area and without their enthusiastic participation in advanced medical management. The only way to obtain this participation, these large numbers, and this kind of enthusiasm is to bring the venture's potential down to the bottom line for physicians, inclusive of a structure of ownership and governance that renders them partners, if not the driving force behind the venture.

Turning to the issue of the relationship between the provider network and the insurance company, there are several different ways to approach a joint venture. The first issue to address is the ownership of the joint venture. Ownership can be viewed with great importance or with little importance, depending on the point of view of providers. For example, if a provider network sees ownership as inextricably linked to governance, the provider network will probably want to have equal ownership with the insurance company. Likewise, if a provider network views a joint venture as some kind of stepping stone wherein the entity will ultimately be sold for what could be a large return on investment, the provider network is going to be most interested in owning as much as possible of the joint venture on a parity basis with the insurance company.

On the other hand, not-for-profit community hospitals and community-based physicians that are interested more in the ongoing financial potential of managing care as well as the potential of increasing market position may not be as interested in outright ownership as they are in issues of governance and operations. As long as providers are able to govern their affairs to their satisfaction and participate in bonus pools, premiums, and other revenues to their satisfaction, issues of who owns stock in the joint venture, how that stock may be divided, or even what kind of entity the joint venture is may not be of major concern. As was mentioned previously when discussing physicians, providers in a provider/insurer joint venture need to recognize that the real value to them lies in their ability to free up a greater percentage of premium dollars for bonus pools and profits through advanced medical management.

Very few areas of the United States are highly evolved in terms of HMO penetration with extremely low premiums, and even in those areas there is often a consumer backlash against HMOs. Thus, the costs of engaging in highly evolved managed care and medical management is relatively low compared with the premiums that can be obtained. This is true in both the commercial sector and the Medicare sector. Some analysts believe that the potential of joint ventures that approach Medicare recipients alone is so great that dollars almost beyond imagination can be freed up. Of course, as competition increases and as the consuming market becomes more sophisticated, a certain portion of these windfalls from managed care will disappear, but, even taking this into account, it is expected that highly evolved medical management of consumer-responsive health care insurance products will always yield significant and ongoing positive cash flows. Hence, providers in a provider/insurer joint venture need to position themselves to participate fully in those positive cash flows on an ongoing basis.

What distinguishes joint ventures from full-risk contracting is the presence of an explicit partnership structure with mutually agreed goals and activities along the full continuum of functions, including product development, marketing, pricing, medical management, etc. The degree to which the joint venture will be successful and will benefit providers over and above any kind of full-risk contract hinges on the depth of the partnership attitude on the part of all parties as well as the extent to which a partnership atmosphere is carried through into the detailed implementation of various facets of the overall project.

There are several ways to approach the issue of revenue sharing among the partners of a provider/insurer joint venture. Two broad categories of approach that seem to be common are:

- Revenues are shared first to cover costs, depending on the functions that each party is performing, and the remaining profits are split in some fashion.

- All costs and revenues are lumped and the parties simply agree on a "global split."

The first of these general approaches relies on the assumption that providers and the insurer will divide functions on the basis of the appropriateness of the activity and the relative strengths of each party. For example, the insurance company is often more willing and better able to take on traditional insurance functions such as claims processing, whereas providers take on credentialing, quality assurance, and medical management. When providers take on these functions, they also assume significant additional costs previously borne by the insurer. Providers are, in this instance, entitled to revenues similar to those that might be realized in a full-risk contract with a number of delegated authorities.

It is commonly thought that the universe of premium revenues to be split for administrative overhead and profit are about 25 percent of total premium dollars. In a situation in which providers do not assume any responsibilities other than providing medical care, the insurer would ordinarily receive the full 25 percent, out of which they would allocate money for administrative costs and profit. In joint ventures, however, if providers are performing a number of functions that previously had been performed by the insurer, the insurance company's allocated overhead and profit portion might be reduced to 10 or 15 percent of the premium, with the remainder going to providers. Once the administrative split has been negotiated, the remaining 75 percent of premium dollars is allocated first to actual loss claims, second to the purchase of reinsurance and any other necessary "back stops," and third to bonus pools based on the differential between the total remaining premium dollars and deductions for loss payouts.

Under the second general approach to revenue sharing—the so-called "global" approach—the parties do not necessarily concern themselves with an allocation of costs by function but, rather, draw a circle around the entire joint venture and decide on an overall formula "split." For example, if the parties are 50/50 owners in the venture, they might decide to split all costs and profits down the middle. It is also possible that the parties may decide on different global splits for administrative overhead and medical overhead claims payouts etc. They might decide, for example, to split administrative overhead on a 2/3-1/3 basis, but split medical losses 50/50.

The split of bonus pools from medical management is sometimes tilted in favor of providers in order to entice physicians to enthusiastically participate in the entire project. Keep in mind that, in the traditional insurance business, an insurance company might take 25 percent of the total premium dollar, allocating 15 to 20 percent for administrative overhead and the remainder for profit. In other words, when constructing premium pricing in a traditional insurance scheme, 75 percent or more of the dollars are assumed to be paid out in claims. Thus, in a joint venture, if the insurance company gives providers the majority of bonus pool dollars resulting from medical management—while still building in some profit from the administrative side of its designated activities—the insurance company may still be doing better than it would have otherwise, because "net dollars" are being freed up through the medical management.

Another way of saying this is that advanced medical management is really at the heart of what makes a joint venture between providers and insurance work. The most important parties in terms of implementing the medical management process are physicians, followed by hospitals. Therefore, generation of bonus pool dollars really begins with the process of motivating physicians to focus on the project at hand. If bonus pool dollars are generated, it is because physicians—and, to some extent, hospitals—have earned these dollars through their medical management activities. Hence, if an insurance company can build in some profit margin from administrative activities and also capture at least some of the bonus pool dollars, it comes out ahead even if its portion of the bonus pool on a percentage basis is much less than that of the providers. This becomes even more true if the joint venture also creates net additional market share for all parties.

It bears repeating that the single most crucial element in forging a successful provider/insurer joint venture is the physician component. This is true with respect to both the numbers and the geographic spread of physicians and in terms of obtaining the commitment of physicians to engage in appropriate kinds of advanced medical management. Insurers and hospitals should not even think about a joint venture unless they are willing to recognize and reward the essential role of physicians and, at the same time, accept the fact that very little of the capital will be coming from physicians. The trade-off is that physicians, when properly motivated, will make the entire project successful.

The Establishment or Acquisition of an Insurance Entity by Providers

It is commonly held that the ultimate stage of evolution among health care providers is to become insurers in their own right. Eliminating the so-called insurance "middlemen" is thought to accomplish two significant objectives: first, elimination of or dramatic reduction in layers of interstitial costs and, second, establishment of a more direct relationship between providers and consumers. Theoretically, both of these objectives should be attainable.

Regarding reduction of costs in the system, there is no question that middlemen do take a significant amount of the premium dollar for administration and profit. If providers can establish insurance entities that are specifically set up to break even and not necessarily make a profit on traditional insurance functions, costs could be reduced. In addition, providers who now contract with insurance companies and/or HMOs often duplicate some insurance company functions that both kinds of organizations perform simultaneously. For example, some provider organizations have risk contracts that permit providers to handle such functions as credentialing, quality assurance, and utilization management while, at the same time, the insurance entity is "shadowing" the providers by performing virtually the same functions in order to make certain that providers do their jobs correctly. Many believe that, if providers owned and operated their own insurance entities, there would be no need for these "watch dog" kinds of duplicative efforts and the resultant costs.

Regarding the establishment of a more direct connection between providers and consumers, direct ownership of an insurance entity by providers would appear to have the strong potential to eliminate some of the backlash against managed care that consumers have evidenced in recent years. The thinking here is that, by continuing to have middlemen involved in the health insurance process, providers are continuing to abdicate more and more of the practice of medicine to insurers. The litany of state-by-state anti-HMO initiatives is too lengthy to discuss in detail here, except to say that, during 1996 and 1997, what can only be characterized as a "wave" of anti-HMO legislation permeated some 40 states and, to some extent, Congress. Recent surveys of consumers have revealed that many Americans believe that decisions about their medical care are no longer made by physicians and hospitals but, rather, by business middlemen at insurance organizations that are motivated totally by a high profit and a good return on investment. If middlemen could be taken out of the equation, the theory goes, costs could be reduced, benefits could be increased, and providers would be more responsive to the needs of consumers.

Thus, by virtue of the economics, the politics, the public relations, and the overall "mission" of health care providers, the timing would seem to be perfect for providers to become insurers and contract directly with consumers.

Much legislative and regulatory activity has occurred in this area in the past two years. In addition to passage by Congress of Medicare direct contracting legislation, some states have applied for and received permission from the Health Care Financing Administration (HCFA) to permit Medicaid direct contracting. On the commercial side, a handful of states have either permitted or are about to permit provider networks to "direct contract" with self-insured employers without having to obtain a state insurance license. Many other states are considering measures designed to make it easier for providers to obtain insurance licenses and to capitalize and/or acquire insurance companies.

It is possible, if "direct contracting" becomes widespread, that provider networks will not have to acquire or start their own insurance companies; they will be de facto provider/insurers without actually owning an insurance company. Nonetheless, because of the regulatory and legislative complexities—to say nothing of the formidable lobbying muscle of the insurance industry—it is expected to take several years for direct contracting to flourish.

Therefore, a number of providers have decided not to wait for permissive direct contracting legislation and have formed and are forming licensed insurance entities. These entities can be divided into the following types of configurations:

- HMOs that are new start-ups by physicians and are physician-owned.

- HMOs and insurance companies that are new start-ups by hospitals and/or hospital networks.

- HMOs and insurance companies that are acquired by physicians and in which the underlying insurance entity existed prior to the acquisition as a viable, state-licensed entity.

- HMOs and insurance companies that are acquired by hospitals and/or hospital networks and that existed as viable, state-licensed entities prior to the acquisition.

- Joint start-up or acquisition of insurance entities by hospitals and physicians—and in some cases other types of investors—acting in concert.

To date, the degree of success of these kinds of efforts varies widely, and a number of them have fallen significantly short of their potential or original vision. However, these efforts are all worth studying, for it is important to understand possible shortcomings and, in so doing, better comprehend the scope of challenges involved in the start up or acquisition of an insurance entity by a provider network.

Perhaps the most important place to start this particular discussion is to explore what is meant by "provider network" in these various configurations and how the creation of the provider network can have a far-reaching impact on the success of the entire project.

Both the scope and the composition of a provider network in the context of insurance company formation are critical factors that, in this author's view, are so important as to be predetermining.

- In terms of scope, it appears that a provider network needs to be large enough to offer a comprehensive array of medical services over a large geographic and population catchment area. Just as insurance companies that are marketing to a given region feel compelled to sign up providers from throughout the region, so should a provider network include network members that can bring to the network comprehensiveness of service while covering the geography.

- Marketing to an entire region (with "region" here defined as an SMSA, state, or other regionally defined market penetration area) is too expensive not to spread marketing costs over many providers in a provider/insurer configuration. This is a straightforward financial reason for the provider network to be large and to cover the region's geography and population.

- Whether contractually or through direct membership, the scope of a provider network that is going to become an insurer needs to include tertiary care, home care, rehabilitation medicine, and other kinds of medical services that would be covered by a complete health insurance policy held by a consumer.

- In terms of the composition of the provider network, early indications are that neither hospitals nor physicians acting alone can become successful provider/insurers. In most cases of physician insurance company or HMO formation, physicians have not been able to raise the necessary capital. In addition, physicians face a built-in public relations problem when they attempt to act as a physician-only network; the efforts run the risk of being viewed by the public as some kind of scheme for the physicians to make more money. Hospital-driven provider/insurer networks, on the other hand, are rarely able to gain the trust of enough physicians to make their network a regional presence, much less make the physicians enthusiastic about conducting the kinds of medical management and marketing efforts that are essential to success.

Although hospitals do, theoretically, have the capital to form a provider/insurer entity, they are wasting precious capital as long as physicians remain skeptical of, or even antagonistic toward, a hospital-owned insurance entity. A provider configuration in which hospitals and physicians can come to some partnership arrangement prior to forming or acquiring an insurance entity appears to be the approach with the highest probability of success.

Once the not insignificant issues of scope and configuration are addressed, a major question becomes: Do providers start a new insurance company or acquire an existing company? (It should be pointed out that even addressing this question presupposes that a favorable kind of joint venture with an existing insurance company has been evaluated and ruled out.) Some factors influencing this important "make or buy" decision are:

- A detailed market assessment needs to be conducted to measure the relative market share of all existing insurance companies and/or HMOs in the market. This would include, of course, identification of any other provider-owned insurance entities, including those in the start-up phase.

- Assessment of insurance entities in the market should include identification of relative market position, marketing strengths and weaknesses, market segments to which the entity sells its insurance products, specific insurance products, relative pricing of each product, marketing approach, infrastructure, and any known expansion plans.

- Any existing joint venture arrangements between provider networks and insurers should be identified and described.

- A matrix should be created by major market segment listing existing players and describing existing market penetration. The major market segments in this matrix are Medicare, Medicaid, self-insured employers, commercial HMOs and commercial indemnity insurers/PPOs. If possible, the size of each market segment in terms of population should be identified.

- An "opportunity prioritization" should be constructed, indicating which of the above market segments should be focused on and why. Where possible, geography and population should be described and evaluated from the perspective of the provider network's market penetration potential.

- Provider-owned HMOs and insurance entities should be looked at carefully to evaluate whether acquisition or merger is feasible and whether such a move is logical, given the market opportunity priorities that the provider network wishes to pursue.

- A start-up budget and timetable should be prepared for creating and licensing a new insurance entity to address whatever market or markets are deemed to be high priority.

- The start-up program should be compared with acquisition of an existing entity, assuming that such an entity exists in the market and is deemed appropriate, given market priorities.

The cost/benefit analysis involved in the decision to acquire an existing insurance organization or start a new one involves answering several fundamental questions:

- What are the comparative costs in dollars?

- What are the comparative costs in time? For example, an entity that already possesses the necessary insurance and/or HMO licenses has already gone through the sometimes lengthy state regulatory process. Although many states are attempting to streamline the acquisition of insurance licenses by provider networks, this can still be a costly, time-consuming process.

- Are there any existing market presence advantages that an existing insurance entity might have? If so, would the existing entity consider selling, and what would be the cost? (It is important to keep in mind that for-profit companies with stockholders can be expensive to acquire.)

- How much actual insurance and claims experience does the existing insurance entity have?

- How much infrastructure and administrative support does the existing entity have, versus starting an insurer with none of these capabilities in place?

It is difficult to generalize further on these points without knowing the specifics of a given market and circumstances. However, a provider network should carefully examine the possibility of acquiring an existing insurer before concluding that it should start a new insurance entity. Acquisition of an existing insurance entity can be an attractive option, even if that entity is small and relatively inactive, because the organization has gone through the regulatory approval processes. In an era in which both regulatory and business factors are beginning to favor establishment of insurance entities by providers, a savings of time that might otherwise be expended in the regulatory approval stage for a start-up insurer can position the provider network ahead of competitors as long as other insurance business fundamentals are expeditiously addressed.

The first principle to be recognized in a discussion of markets to be served and products to be offered by a provider/insurer network is that both insurance of defined populations and delivery of health care services tend to be regional in nature. National insurers contract on a regional basis and, most often, market regionally. Likewise, provider networks tend to be organized regionally. It is advisable for provider networks to organize and operate, at least initially, on a regional basis for the following reasons:

- As stated above, both the provision of health care and the contracting in health insurance programs tend to be regional.

- Both hospitals and physicians know their regional markets and interact with each other and with their peers in those markets.

- The practical aspects of attending meetings dictate that initial organizing efforts be undertaken among network members within a reasonable geographic radius of driving time.

- Both the business and the medical management aspects of network formation and operation require that network members work closely together and be geographically accessible.

All of this is not to say that a multi-regional or even national provider network is not possible, especially among providers with a common background, philosophy, mission, and governance approach. One obvious example of the potential for some kind of national provider/insurer network would be Catholic hospitals and health systems throughout the United States. These organizations share a common heritage, are all not-for-profit, and are all community service-oriented. It would seem to be feasible for Catholic organizations to put together at least some elements of a national provider/insurer network, even if the elements turned out to be limited to the provision of infrastructure and other technical support services and left other functions, such as marketing, credentialing, quality assurance, and even insurance product design, to regional or super-regional subsets that would have greater latitude in assembling their own types of provider networks, given specific characteristics of respective regional markets.

Even though formation of national organizations of provider/insurers appears to be, in some instances, an attractive and enormously potent possibility, significant political and logistical barriers exist. Regional provider/insurer networks are much more likely to form initially, perhaps later on linking together on a super-regional or national scale. The important goal from the perspective of providers is to encompass a region that is large enough to make the effort worthwhile and, at the same time, be geographically able to facilitate logistical and organizational efforts to make the entire project able to be accomplished within a reasonable time.

It is highly unlikely that a provider network will be able to start out from day one with a full complement of members, even if the network is strictly regional. As with any other new type of enterprise or joint venture, initial provider membership may constitute a percentage of what is ultimately desired. Health care providers that envision building a regional provider/insurer network are well advised to begin with the philosophy that a limited number of their counterparts will become the founding members and lead early organizational and planning efforts. The goal of the founders should be to educate and communicate enthusiasm to others, continually recruiting new members until the membership achieves critical mass, if not full maturity.

Providers wishing to establish a provider/insurer network should not be discouraged by the relative degree of managed care penetration in their region, even if the region has a high percentage of HMO capitated-type penetration. There is no market in the United States that is impervious to or insulated from the entry of a new provider/insurer, as long as the provider/insurer network is structured properly and is consumer-friendly. A highly evolved managed care market could actually be a good place to start a provider/insurer network, as long as the network's insurance benefits are consumer-friendly, cost-effective, and comprehensive. If these elements are in place and if the provider/insurer network is able to cultivate a good general image and to differentiate itself and its products in the market, the presence of HMOs and large insurance companies should not be intimidating.

The two most important policy decisions on the part of a provider network that wishes to become a provider/insurer are identifying the specific segments of the consumer population to whom products will be offered and designing the insurance products. With the passage of Section 4001 of the Balanced Budget Act of 1997, which contains the Medicare+Choice Program, the Medicare population could be considered a good market to which a provider/insurer network should initially focus its efforts. There are several reasons why focusing on the Medicare population could be advantageous:

- With passage of the new legislation, Congress has, in effect, given its blessing to the concept of direct contracting in the Medicare program. Accompanying this will be development of national standards by HCFA that will, ideally, result in guidance to provider/insurer networks.

- From a marketing and public relations point of view, the elderly are more likely than many other groups to be skeptical of HMOs and managed care in general. This skepticism can be converted into a potent marketing advantage by a provider/insurer network, especially if the network is not-for-profit, community service-oriented, and consumer-friendly.

- By focusing on the Medicare population, a provider/insurer network does not need to be all-encompassing regionally. Such a network can effectively serve the Medicare population even if there are significant gaps in geographic and population coverage. Most of the Medicare population is retired, so that every hospital has within its natural service area a number of Medicare recipients who stay in that area and are not commuting to work or engaging in other activities that affect the younger, commercially insured population. It is quite possible, therefore, for a provider/insurer network to begin its activities by serving its Medicare population, even though more hospital members of a regional network may ultimately be desired. This feature of the Medicare population has the practical effect of improving organizational logistics and reducing the start-up time of a provider/insurer network.

● Marketing to the Medicare population can be accomplished less expensively than marketing to the general commercial population.

Some provider/insurer networks are also targeting the Medicaid population for many of the same reasons outlined above. Medicaid recipients tend to reside in or near natural hospital service area boundaries. Many states are encouraging development by providers of Medicaid managed care programs and products. If the underlying reimbursement is structured properly and is accompanied by other reasonable features, a provider-sponsored Medicaid program can be successful.

Serving the commercial markets presents different and, some would say, much greater challenges than attempting to serve the Medicare or Medicaid markets. One hurdle that providers face when confronting the commercial sector is establishment of a more geographically comprehensive provider network than would otherwise be the case. Unlike Medicare or Medicaid markets, the population to be served for the commercial sector does not usually correspond to natural hospital service areas. For example, just because a company is located within a hospital's service area does not mean that employees and their families reside in that service area; as a matter of fact, this is rarely the case. Hence, while a provider network may be marketing to businesses that are headquartered in specific locations, employees of those businesses may live quite some distance away, necessitating that physicians and hospital be located disparately from the headquarters of the company to whom the hospital in question may be marketing.

In short, provider networks that intend to develop and market insurance products to a commercially insured population need to be much more comprehensive in scope and in membership, both with respect to hospitals and medical practices. Whereas, with the Medicare population, a network can start with an initial provider membership that may not include every area of a region, this is not the case in a competitive, commercially oriented network. In order to market commercial health insurance products to even one sizable corporation, the network needs to cover the entire geography and population in a given region almost from day one.

The practical effect of all of this is that provider networks just starting out are probably well advised not to tackle the commercial sector unless they are able to cover the regional geography and population from the beginning, as may be the case in medium-sized or smaller markets. It is much more practical for provider/insurer networks to focus on the Medicare and Medicaid populations while, at the same time, building up the underlying membership in the provider network so that it does become regional. Then the provider/insurer can start with self-insured employers and other targeted populations. One needs to keep in mind that, during the time such a provider network is building up its membership, it is also in a position to accumulate capital for marketing expenses, which should not be underestimated, particularly when marketing to the commercially insured population. Any provider network that intends to do this must recognize that the existing insurance companies and HMOs are not going to sit by and permit the new provider/insurer network to take away their subscribers. In the commercial sector, an expensive marketing campaign is much more likely to occur for this reason.

This is not to say that marketing to the Medicare sector is easy. Many established insurance companies and HMOs already have products designed to target the Medicare population. A provider/insurer network that focuses on this market is certainly not guaranteed success. Increasingly, commercial insurers and established HMOs are creating Medicare managed care products that are considered to be more consumer-friendly. Now that Congress has officially set in motion the permissibility of Medicare direct contracting by providers, existing insurers and HMOs are not likely to wait around for new provider/insurer networks to encroach on their markets.

From an overall marketing point of view, it is vital that would-be provider/insurers keep two primary objectives in mind:

- Establishment of a strong, consumer-friendly image.

- Creation of insurance products that are significantly differentiated from other insurance products in the market.

It is the presence of both of these key elements—among others but above all others—that gives the provider/insurer the highest likelihood of success. These two crucial elements absolutely go together; a provider/insurer network that has a good public image but has inadequate products is going to fail, as will a network that has good products but does not have a positive public image.

Above all else, health care providers need to make certain that they avoid doing anything that is associated with the negative perceptions on the part of the general public about managed care. In addition, everything must be done to create the impression that the concept of a provider-owned health insurance entity is beneficial to consumers and is not some kind of scheme to enrich providers at the expense of consumers or to take managed care service shortcuts at the consumers' expense.

As important as it is to design health insurance packages that consumers want, it is just as important to avoid features that consumers find irritating, inconvenient, or outright unacceptable. Some of these negative features include restrictions on choice of primary care physician, undue restrictions on the ability of primary care physicians to refer to specialists, restrictions on the ability of patients to discuss program costs and treatment costs with physicians, and restrictions on the ability of physicians to discuss treatment options with patients and to refer patients to specialists who might be "outside the plan." Prospective provider/insurers need to be at least as responsive to avoiding or minimizing these negative features of health plans as they are to designing the positive features of their products.

It is not enough for a provider/insurer to offer one more managed care program that contains all of the negative features now present in the traditional insurance industry, even if the new program can be brought in at a lower premium dollar. Consumers are ever more conscious about the downside of HMOs and other managed care programs, and they are becoming more sophisticated about measuring the tradeoffs among cost, access, and price. If a provider network can offer health insurance products designed around meeting the positive needs of consumers and avoiding the negative concerns, the sophisticated provider/insurer will have accomplished a goal that will singularly differentiate it from all other traditional insurers—creating products that have higher value, keeping in mind all of the elements that constitute value.

Sorting It All Out: The Leadership Challenge for Physician Executives

Regardless which type of configuration a provider network has or where the network is positioned on the "continuum of risk," physician executives face some formidable challenges that can be divided into three leadership areas:

- Physician-to-physician leadership—convincing colleagues to embrace the right kind of highly evolved managed care and to actively participate in reengineering of medical delivery.

- Physician-to-hospital leadership—working with hospitals and hospital networks to create structures and arrangements that permit providers to jointly move up the continuum of risk.

- Management leadership—creating and managing the vital underlying administrative/infrastructure underpinnings that give physicians and other caregivers the tools to "manage" care in a consumer-friendly manner.

Above all else, the physician leader understands that physicians possess the most precious asset of all: the physician-patient relationship, the personal relationship, the one-on-one human service of compassion and competence that is the essence of what is good in our health care system. Physicians need to take the leadership to create new structures for caregivers who are able to function in a system that permits them to care.

References

1. The author expresses appreciation to Mr. Ed Hirshfeld, Vice President, Health Law, and Kathy Nino, Staff Attorney, of the American Medical Association for providing a summary of the key features of the Balanced Budget Act of 1997 affecting Medicare Part C.
2. Excerpted from the American Medical Association's summary of certain provisions of the Balanced Budget Act of 1997; "Provider Sponsored Organization Provisions In The Balance Budget Act of 1997", American Medical Association, Office of the General Counsel, Aug. 6, 1997.
3. This section, running to the last section of the chapter, is excerpted with permission from Unland, J., "The Range of Provider/Insurer Configurations." *Journal of Health Care Finance* 24(2):1-35, Winter 1998.

Chapter 19

An Annotated Bibliography for Physician Executives

Arthur Lazarus, MD, MBA

The topic of medical management has received much attention in both the lay press and the scientific literature, yet there is no central well-organized repository of information on this topic except in a few books. The interested reader must comb the literature and at best can obtain information in piecemeal fashion based largely on limited anecdotal experiences. It was with this in mind that I undertook the task of compiling a bibliography for and about physician executives.

I searched the MEDLINE and Health Planning and Administration databases using the keywords "physician executive" and "physician manager." I then searched bibliographies of articles retrieved by the computerized search. Both searches revealed articles that were objective and contemporary and that provided insight into the changing role of physician executives in health care organizations. I selected a total of 14 publications for this bibliography, nine of which report results of original research.

No claim has been made that this list is definitive or all-inclusive. I devised it primarily for health care professionals—physician executives as well as nonphysician managers—hoping that it would be a useful guide and would stimulate additional reading. A bibliography such as this must be updated as newer research and perspectives change the nature and scope of physician executive responsibilities.

History and Overview

Hodge, R., and Nash, D. "The Physician-Executive." In *Future Practice Alternatives in Medicine*, Second edition, Nash, D., Editor. New York, N.Y.: Igaku-Shoin, 1993.

This chapter is an expansion and update of an article that appeared in the *New England Journal of Medicine* in 1986. Written by two physician executives—the Vice President of a large health care system and Director of a center for health policy and clinical outcomes—it provides a personal perspective of health care management, traces the history and development of medical management, and discusses how physicians who aspire to the upper echelons of management can obtain the necessary skills. The authors make the point that medical administration is the equivalent of a board certifiable specialty.

Managed Care

Schneller, E. "The Leadership and Executive Potential of Physicians in an Era of Managed Care Systems." *Hospital and Health Services Administration* 36(1):43-55, Spring 1991.

Involvement of physicians in management is not a new phenomenon in American medicine. What is different is that an increased number of physicians are employees of organizations and that "maintaining the integrity of managed care systems requires an administrative response qualitatively different from previous attempts to shape the delivery of services." Employment of physician executives is a visible part of that response. Physician executives ensure the clinical integrity of health care organizations, determine the structure of health care benefits, present quality assurance data and other information to the public, accredit providers for cost-effective treatment, and design systems of care. Physician executives, however, risk losing the loyalty of other physicians if they become overly identified with business executives.

Relationships with Lay Managers

O'Connor, P., and Shewchuk, R. "Enhancing Administrator-Clinician Relationships: The Role of Psychological Type." *Health Care Management Review* 18(2):57-65, Spring 1993.

Relations between physicians and administrators have been fraught with conflict for most of this century. O'Connor and Shewchuk studied psychological differences between physicians and administrators using the Myers-Briggs Type Indicator (MBTI), a widely used personality assessment. Physicians and administrators tend to be polar opposites. The latter are extraverted, sensing, thinking, and judging, whereas physicians tend to be introverted, intuitive, feeling, and perceiving. Only by understanding and appreciating these differences can physicians and administrators communicate effectively and avoid conflict.

Management Style

Wilson, A., and Schroeder, N. "Physician and Nonphysician Managers as Decision Makers: Are the Differences Justified or Just an Illusion." *Physician Executive* 18(5):3-6, Sept.-Oct. 1992.

Four different models of decision making were examined in 423 physician executives and nonphysician managers. Physician managers tend to be "political" in their decision making, i.e., likely to negotiate to attain specific goals. Nonphysician managers are swayed more by fiscal concerns. When various decision-making styles were rank ordered according to the likelihood of using those styles, both physicians and nonphysician managers showed similar tendencies. Physician executives are able to correctly identify an appropriate decision style for a strategic decision.

Professional Development

Silver, M., and others. "Critical Factors in the Professional Development of the Psychiatrist-Administrator." *Hospital and Community Psychiatry* 41(1):71-4, Jan. 1990.

Two hundred and forty-four psychiatrist executives from the metropolitan New York City area were surveyed. The process of becoming a physician executive is complex and involves the interplay of at least five factors: personality traits, clinical training, formal training in administration, administrative experience, and a mentor relationship. Respondents felt there was a discrepancy between their actual and their ideal experiences in the areas of the mentor relationship and formal administrative training. These issues need to be addressed further in medical school and residency training.

Career Paths

Kindig, D., and others. "Career Paths of Physician Executives." *Health Care Management Review* 16(4):11-20, Fall 1991.

Nearly 900 physician executives were surveyed. Forty percent of physicians had held administrative positions in more than one type of health care organization. Senior physician executives held four or more positions in a single type of organization or two positions in different types of organizations. Time spent in administration increased with age and years in administration. Senior physician executives spent less then 10 percent of their time in direct patient care. Advancement to executive positions requires flexibility and willingness to move between organizations and across organizational types.

The Glass Ceiling

Tesch, B., and others. "Promotion of Women Physicians in Academic Medicine: Glass Ceiling or Sticky Floor?" JAMA 273(13):1022-5, April 5, 1995.

The glass ceiling refers to barriers that prevent professionals from achieving senior-level positions. These barriers are invisible yet impassable. The careers of minority and female physician executives have been affected by the glass ceiling. Female physicians in academic medical centers are promoted more slowly than their male counterparts. This finding cannot be explained by productivity or by differential attrition from academic medicine. The slower promotion of women faculty appears to be due to gender bias, however unintended.

Organizational Roles

Dunham, N., and others. "The Value of the Physician Executive Role to Organizational Effectiveness and Performance." *Health Care Management Review* 19(4):56-63, Fall 1994.

Physician executives perform many administrative functions outside the clinical arena. Such "boundary-spanning" roles include financial planning, capital budgeting, technology assessment, cost-benefit analysis, marketing, and recruiting. These areas have not previously been viewed as major physician executive functions. Ironically, compared with other managers, physician executives underrate the value of these functions to their organizations. Physician executives should assist with these activities because nonmedical managers deem them important.

Practice Versus Administration

Weiner, L. "Part-Time Medical Director: Way Station or End of the Line?" *Physician Executive* 20(3):12-5, March 1994.
As medical management becomes more complex and specialized, physicians interested in the field must be identified, nurtured, and properly trained. Although managing and practicing are not mutually exclusive, the demands of each make it difficult to do both. Administrators erroneously believe it is necessary for physician executives to maintain clinical practices. Physicians who wear the hat of part-time medical director unwittingly play to a naive management team that fails to recognize the potential of physician executives. Part-time medical directors are often sequestered and given limited duties. If full-time management is the ultimate goal, physicians should consider immersing themselves in it at the outset.

Training and Education

Lloyd, J., and Lyons, M. "The Physician Executive 'Arrives'—A New Generation Prepares for the Future." *Physician Executive* 21(1):22-6, Jan. 1995.

According to a survey of physicians of the American College of Physician Executives, 9.4 percent of physician executives have MBA degrees and another 38 percent are working on MBAs or intend to do so. Other physicians are pursuing traditional health care administration degrees, law degrees, or other academic credentials. Formal education past medical school is not mandatory for physician executives, but experience alone may not be sufficient for advancement in a management career. Apart from attending graduate schools of business administration or health care administration, seminars, workshops, and other types of educational programs are available and should be considered.

Compensation

Physician Executive Compensation Survey. Sponsored by the American College of Physician Executives and conducted by Cjeka and Company, 1997.

Data were obtained from more than 3,912 physician executives. Median total compensation (salary plus bonus and incentive) was $188,850 for all physicians executives. Median total compensation for physicians spending 100% of their time in management was $166,000. Compensation was influenced by management experience, title or function, additional postgraduate degrees, industry sector or type of organization, medical specialty, and geographic location.

Physician Executive Compensation Report: A 1995-96 Survey and Ten-Year Trends. Tampa, Fla.: Physician Executive Management Center, 1996

This survey, conducted annually, was based on responses from 375 physician executives in hospitals, group practices, and managed care organizations. Average total compensation for all participants was $183,732. This is an increase of more than 5 percent in one year and about 16 percent in two years. Physician executives report an increase in job scope and responsibilities as a result of managed care. Virtually all physician executives were satisfied with their decision to become managers and recommended similar career direction to their physician colleagues. By all accounts, physician executives are well compensated for their efforts.

Portents for Management

Smallwood, K., and Wilson, N. "Physician Executives Past, Present, and Future." *Southern Medical Journal* 85(8):840-4, Aug. 1992.

In the future, the demand for physician executives will increase dramatically. Nonmedical health care executives, however, may oppose the development of physician executives. Furthermore, physician executives must answer to physicians who claim they (physician executives) have "joined the suits." Despite these difficulties, physicians appear to be rising to meet the challenges of managing the medical-industrial complex.